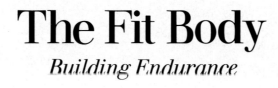

The Fit Body
Building Endurance

Fitness, Health & Nutrition was created by Rebus, Inc. and published by Time-Life Books.

REBUS, INC.

Publisher: RODNEY FRIEDMAN

Editor: CHARLES L. MEE JR.
Senior Editor: THOMAS DICKEY
Managing Editor: SUSAN BRONSON
Senior Writer: WILLIAM DUNNETT
Associate Editors: NONA CLELAND,
CAMILLE CUSUMANO, CARL LOWE

Art Director: ROBBIN SCHIFF
Designer: DEBORAH RAGASTO
Photographer: STEVEN MAYS
Photo Stylist: NOLA LOPEZ
Picture Editor: DEBORAH BULL

Recipe Editor: BONNIE J. SLOTNICK
Test Kitchen Director: MARJORIE QUINCE
Consulting Editor: MARYA DALRYMPLE
Food Consultant: FRAN SHINAGEL
Nutritional Analyst: NANCY MUZECK

Chief of Research: BARBARA JURGENSEN
Assistant Editor: CARNEY MIMMS
Editorial Assistant: JENNIFER MAH

Time-Life Books Inc. is a wholly owned subsidiary of
TIME INCORPORATED

Founder: HENRY R. LUCE 1898-1967

Editor-in-Chief: HENRY ANATOLE GRUNWALD
President: J. RICHARD MUNRO
Chairman of the Board: RALPH P. DAVIDSON
Corporate Editor: RAY CAVE
Group Vice President, Books: REGINALD K. BRACK JR.
Vice President, Books: GEORGE ARTANDI

TIME-LIFE BOOKS INC.

Editor: GEORGE CONSTABLE

Director of Design: LOUIS KLEIN
Director of Editorial Resources: PHYLLIS K. WISE
Acting Text Director: ELLEN PHILLIPS
Editorial Board: RUSSELL B. ADAMS JR., DALE M. BROWN,
ROBERTA CONLAN, THOMAS H. FLAHERTY, DONIA ANN
STEELE, ROSALIND STUBENBERG, KIT VAN TULLEKEN,
HENRY WOODHEAD
Director of Photography and Research: JOHN CONRAD WEISER

President: REGINALD K. BRACK JR.
Executive Vice Presidents: JOHN M. FAHEY JR.,
CHRISTOPHER T. LINEN
Senior Vice Presidents: JAMES L. MERCER,
LEOPOLDO TORALBALLA
Vice Presidents: STEPHEN L. BAIR, RALPH J. CUOMO,
NEAL GOFF, STEPHEN L. GOLDSTEIN, JUANITA T. JAMES,
HALLETT JOHNSON III, ROBERT H. SMITH, PAUL R. STEWART
Director of Production Services: ROBERT J. PASSANTINO

Editorial Operations
Copy Chief: DIANE ULLIUS
Editorial Operations: CAROLINE A. BOUBIN (MANAGER)
Production: CELIA BEATTIE
Library: LOUISE D. FORSTALL

FITNESS, HEALTH & NUTRITION

Building Endurance
Aerobic Workouts

Time-Life Books, Alexandria, Virginia

CONSULTANTS FOR THIS BOOK

For information about any Time-Life book please write:
Reader Information
Time-Life Books
541 North Fairbanks Court
Chicago
Illinois 60611

© 1987 Time-Life Books Inc. All rights reserved. No part of this book may be reproduced in any form or by any electronic or mechanical means, including information storage and retrieval devices or systems, without prior written permission from the publisher except that brief passages may be quoted for reviews. First printing.
Published simultaneously in Canada.
School and library distribution by Silver Burdett Company, Morristown, New Jersey.

TIME-LIFE is a trademark of Time Incorporated U.S.A.

Library of Congress Cataloging-in-Publication Data
The Fit body.
(Fitness, health, and nutrition)
Includes index.
1. Heart. 2. Exercise—Physiological effect.
3. Physical fitness. I. Time-Life Books. II. Series.
[DNLM: 1. Exertion—popular works.
2. Physical Endurance—popular works.
3. Physical Fitness—popular works.
QT 255 F544]
QP114.E9F58 1987   613.7'1   86-23079
ISBN 0-8094-6154-4
ISBN 0-8094-6155-2 (lib. bdg.)

This book is not intended as a medical guide or a substitute for the advice of a physician. Readers, especially those who have or suspect they may have specific medical problems, are urged to consult a physician before beginning any program of strenuous physical exercise.

CONTENTS

Chapter One

ENDURANCE   6

Aerobic endurance: getting it and keeping it, designing your own
program, choosing an exercise and staying with it,
warming up and cooling down

Chapter Two

WALKING   30

Correct posture, striding, race walking, weight-loading

Chapter Three

AEROBIC MOVEMENT   42

Full-body workout, low-impact aerobics, jumping rope,
the right shoes, music for movement

Chapter Four

RUNNING   58

Carriage and alignment, fluid replacement, runner's high, anatomy
of a running shoe, common injuries and how to avoid them

Chapter Five

CYCLING   74

Bicycle touring, cadence, pedaling, taking hills, finding the right bike

Chapter Six

SWIMMING   86

The right stroke, interval training, pyramids, the S curve,
swimmers' ailments, equipment

Chapter Seven

CROSS-COUNTRY SKIING   100

Diagonal stride, double poling, the new skating technique

Chapter Eight

ROWING   114

Cruising, keeping your balance, the right rowing shell,
power pieces, stroke rating

Chapter Nine

CARBOHYDRATES   124

Eating for endurance, the carbo-loading debate, the best
sources, good-tasting and easy-to-make recipes

Acknowledgments   142

Index   143

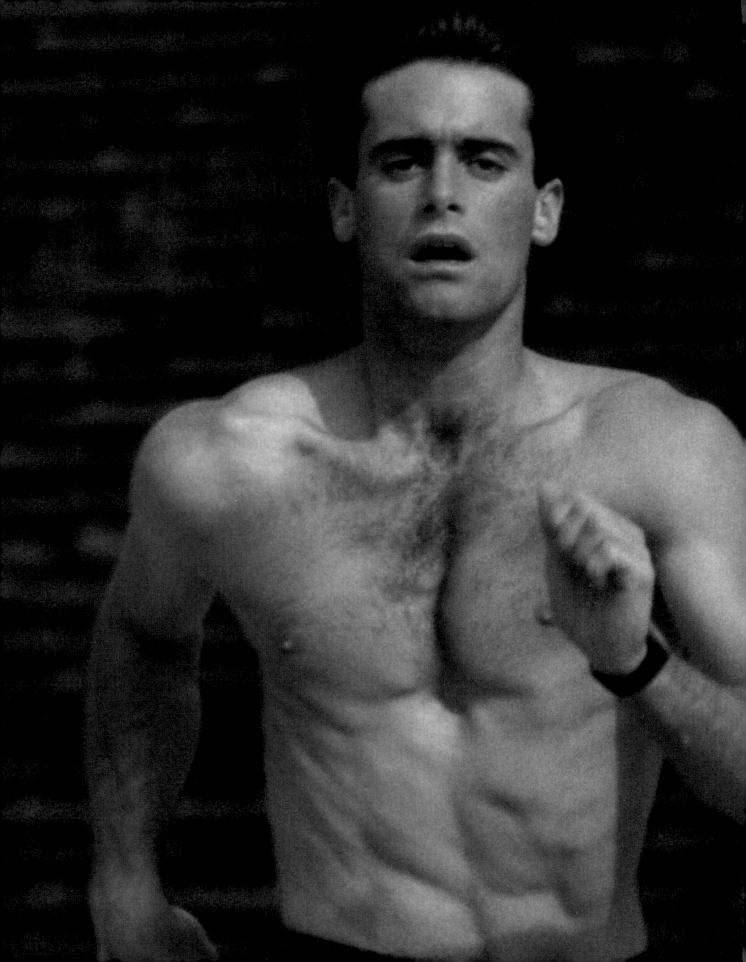

CHAPTER ONE

Endurance

The basic element of fitness: building up the heart and lungs

Of all the elements of fitness, the most crucial is that of cardiovascular endurance — the sustained ability of the heart and lungs and blood to take oxygen from the air and deliver it throughout the body. Every cell in the body requires oxygen to function. The stronger the heart and the more elastic the lungs, the better the cardiovascular system delivers oxygen. And the better the cardiovascular system works, the livelier we feel, the sharper our minds are and the greater the likelihood that we will find ourselves with reserves of energy at the end of the day.

How is endurance built?
Since there is no way to exercise the heart and lungs and blood vessels directly, you must do an exercise that places a demand on the cardiovascular system — an exercise that summons large quantities of oxygen into the system.

In essence, any form of exercise that lasts more than 90 seconds

Fitness and Resting Heart Rate

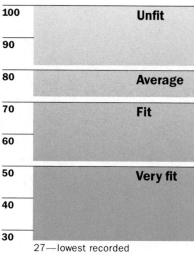

Heartbeats per minute

100	**Unfit**
90	
80	**Average**
70	**Fit**
60	
50	**Very fit**
40	
30	

27—lowest recorded
(in a cross-country skier)

A fit heart pumps more blood with each beat than an unfit heart and so needs to beat fewer times to deliver the oxygen and nutrients the body requires. People who are fit tend to have low resting heart rates; in fact, many endurance athletes have resting heart rates below 50 beats per minute. By contrast, an unfit person's heart rate may be well above 80.

increases fresh supplies of oxygen and is called "aerobic," a word derived from two Greek words meaning "life" and "air." Any exercise that lasts less than 90 seconds, such as lifting weights or jumping a fence, needs almost no fresh oxygen and so is called "anaerobic," or "life" and "no air."

To give your cardiovascular system a thorough enough workout to achieve significant benefits, you must sustain exercise for at least 20 minutes. The exercise should use the large muscle groups like the legs or the arms and shoulders in order to place a substantial demand on the cardiovascular system. The exercise should also be continuous, to keep the oxygen pumping through the system.

The best aerobic exercises are brisk walking, distance running, swimming, cycling, aerobic movement, cross-country skiing, rowing and jumping rope. Exercises like sit-ups, push-ups and other calisthenics, or such start-and-stop sports as volleyball and baseball, may build strength or coordination, but they offer little or no aerobic benefit, even when performed vigorously. Brisk gym workouts on strength-training machines can raise the heart rate, but because their duration is often short and because many of the exercises work smaller muscles, they do not significantly affect the body's intake and delivery of oxygen.

What does an exercise actually do?

Physiologically, your body undergoes an adaptive response to the demands of repeated aerobic exercise. Your heart needs to pump more blood with each beat; with exercise, it becomes stronger and may actually grow larger to do so. Your arteries become dilated so that more blood can be carried to the muscles. The greater blood volume induces capillary formation so that the muscles are better supplied with blood. The muscles themselves become more efficient at absorbing oxygen from the blood and at converting stored carbohydrates and fats into energy. We refer to these changes collectively as "the training effect."

How much exercise must a person do?

To achieve aerobic benefits you must exercise at least three times a week, for 30 minutes each time — five minutes of warm-up to get your heart rate elevated gradually, 20 minutes of aerobic workout called the training phase and five minutes of cool-down to bring your heart rate down gently. Less than this will not help you achieve an adequate training effect, though *any* exercise is better than none.

How will you know when you are fit?

One of the first noticeable indications of improved fitness is that you will have a lower heart rate when you are at rest (your "resting heart rate") than you did before you began an exercise program. In other words, your heart is processing the same amount of blood with less effort than it did before you exercised regularly.

A conditioned person's heart, beating 45 to 50 times a minute at rest, pumps the same amount of blood as does an unconditioned person's

How Exercise Affects the Cardiovascular System

Aerobic exercise makes dramatic demands on the heart and lungs to deliver oxygen throughout the body. The cardiovascular system of a man at rest *(below left)* processes 5,900 milliliters of blood per minute, but during maximal exertion *(below right)*, the man's system processes 24,000 milliliters of blood per minute. The working muscles account for this increased demand: They take up 87 percent of the blood flow during exercise, making the heart beat more often and pump about twice as much blood with each beat.

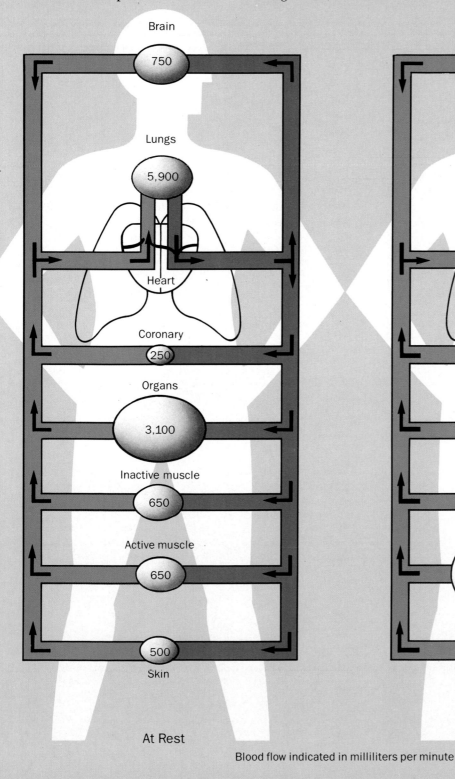

At Rest

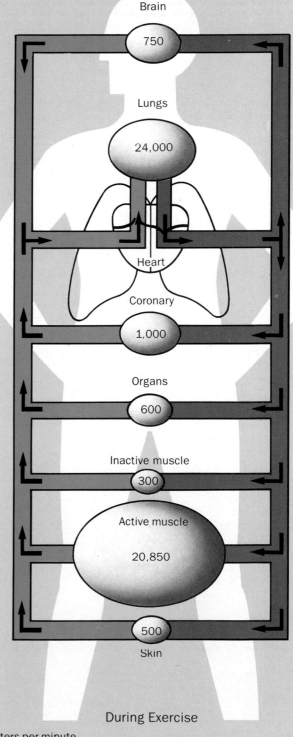

During Exercise

Blood flow indicated in milliliters per minute

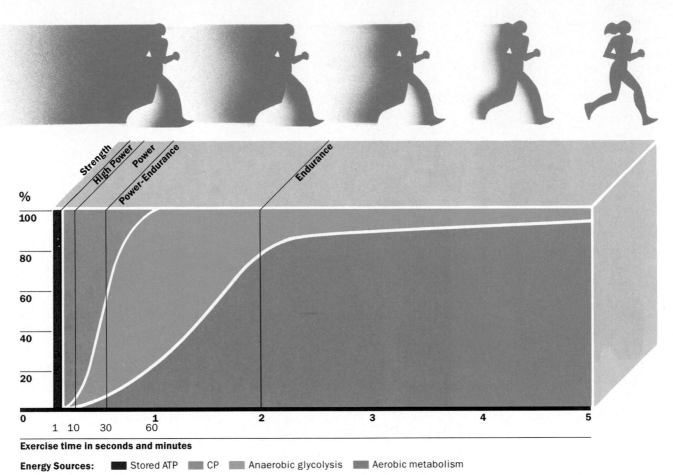

%

100
80
60
40
20
0

Strength
High Power
Power
Power-Endurance
Endurance

1 10 30 1 2 3 4 5
          60

Exercise time in seconds and minutes

Energy Sources: ■ Stored ATP ■ CP ■ Anaerobic glycolysis ■ Aerobic metabolism

The Right Energy System

Food provides our energy, just as gasoline provides energy for an automobile engine. But the engine has only one way of converting fuel, while the body can shift from one energy system to another — a changeover that is crucial in exercising for endurance.

The chart above shows the primary sources of energy during exercise. During the first minute or two of intense effort, the body draws principally on energy stores located within the muscles themselves. These sources are anaerobic, meaning "life" and "no air," since they make little use of oxygen in producing energy.

First, the muscles tap a substance called adenosine triphosphate, or ATP, the only fuel that can directly power a muscle. The stored supply of ATP is minuscule and burns out in about a second. Another phosphate

compound in the muscle — creatine phosphate, or CP — is used to synthesize a fresh supply of ATP. This yields energy for less than 10 seconds of all-out exertion. After that, the muscles begin using a third energy source, glycogen, converted from the glucose in sugars and starches. Muscle glycogen is broken down and refined into ATP during a process called anaerobic glycolysis, which supplies quick energy. But the energy runs out rapidly, mainly because of a by-product called lactic acid that accumulates in muscles and causes them to fatigue.

Meanwhile, the heart and lungs have been getting energy aerobically, or with oxygen. For an activity to last more than a few minutes, this aerobic system must contribute an increasing share of energy to the muscles.

Aerobic metabolism breaks down glycogen into ATP, but without letting harmful by-products build up. This metabolism can also extract energy from fats, which the body stores in far greater abundance than it stores glycogen. The elaborate aerobic system is not able to provide energy nearly as quickly as anaerobic sources, but its contribution is steadier and far more enduring.

The way to keep exercise aerobic is to train continuously but with a less-than-maximum effort. During a workout or a race, bursts of speed may feel exhilarating. But the supply of oxygen cannot meet the suddenly increased energy demands. The muscles shift over to tap anaerobic reserves, and if the surge continues much longer than a minute, the result is certain exhaustion.

heart beating 75 or 80 times a minute. Over the course of a day, the unconditioned person's heart could register 50,000 beats more than the conditioned person's heart. In a year, even taking into account the elevated heart rate for a conditioned person's training sessions, an unconditioned person's heart would beat an "extra" 17 million times. Although no one has proved that a low resting heart rate is good for you (and sometimes a low resting heart rate is simply an individual variation from the norm, a symptom of a low-thyroid condition or certain cardiac disorders), it is most often associated with people who are cardiovascularly fit. Marathon runners frequently report resting heart rates in the low 40s to mid 30s. The lowest recorded resting heart rate, measured in a world-class cross-country skier, is 27 beats per minute.

Is there an exact measurement of fitness?

The most precise determination of fitness is a laboratory test that measures the amount of oxygen someone consumes as he or she runs on a motor-driven treadmill or pedals a stationary bicycle. This measurement is called VO_2max, which refers to the maximum volume of oxygen the body is capable of taking in and using for one minute in the course of intense exercise. (Oxygen is designated "O_2" because it is normally found in a molecule of two atoms.) A high VO_2max is a sign of fitness. The VO_2max values of elite long-distance runners, for example, can be twice those of sedentary individuals.

Although a laboratory test of your VO_2max is the best way to determine your present level of fitness, the step test outlined on pages 20 and 21 is a reliable and safe substitute you can perform at home.

How will endurance make you feel better?

Researchers have consistently found a strong link between regular exercise and "feeling better." This feeling is a series of subtle but significant changes in attitude and mood that seem to occur shortly after the start of an exercise workout and continue for the length of the workout. Explanations for the phenomenon range from the psychochemical (exercise induces the release of morphine-like chemicals in the brain) to the psychological ("I work out, therefore I'm in control of my life").

Whatever the reason, regular exercise seems to stabilize personality. Psychological tests have shown that those who start exercising become more self-confident and optimistic. Furthermore, exercisers have fewer than average symptoms of common mental disorders such as helplessness, anxiety and withdrawal. One study found that a 12-week exercise program was equal to or even better than traditional psychotherapy or antidepressive drugs in treating mild depression. In addition, exercise is more effective than some of the most commonly prescribed tranquilizers in reducing muscle tension.

Exercise evidently helps you handle stress, too. Another study — all but fiendish in its approach — compared two groups of students, one of which participated in a 14-week aerobic exercise program. When

Exercise, Reaction Time and Age

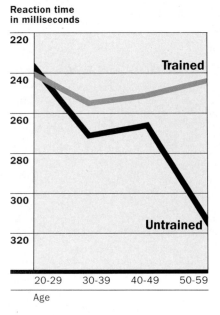

Reaction time in milliseconds

220
240
260
280
300
320

Trained

Untrained

20-29   30-39   40-49   50-59

Age

Aging can slow a person's ability to react quickly, but, according to one study, this is less likely to occur if a person exercises. The study tested 64 men and women, ages 23 to 59, for their reaction time. Half the subjects were serious runners; the other half did not exercise. Among the sedentary group, reaction time — the time required to release a switch on cue — of the older subjects was nearly 50 percent slower than that of the younger subjects, but reaction time of runners remained about the same, regardless of their age.

the exercise program ended, each group took a test. Unaware that most of the problems could not be solved, both groups were informed that the test results would indicate how well they would perform in college. After telling the students of their poor test scores, the scientists found that those without aerobic conditioning had elevated blood pressure, muscle tension and anxiety. The conditioned group displayed lower levels of muscle tension and anxiety, and no elevation in blood pressure.

If you stop exercising, will your muscle turn to fat?
Nothing will change muscle to fat or fat to muscle. Fat and muscle are two different kinds of tissue. Aerobic exercise burns away fat and builds up muscle. If you stop exercising and maintain the same caloric intake, your muscles will weaken and diminish in size, and excess calories will be stored as fat.

Is dieting better than exercise for losing weight?
Although an estimated 65 million Americans are on a diet at any given time, research has shown that dieting alone will not help most of them lose weight. Almost everyone who goes on a weight-reduction diet eventually quits — and regains the lost weight. What is worse, the regained weight often has a higher proportion of fat to muscle than the weight previously lost.

About a third of the weight lost from all types of diets conducted without exercise is lean tissue, not fat tissue. But when you put the weight back on, you will gain back mostly fat tissue, not lean tissue, if you have not been exercising. Going on and off diets constantly over a period of time can make you progressively weaker and, in terms of fat-to-muscle ratio, "fatter."

In any case, exercise alone is more effective than diet alone for weight reduction. Researchers have found that exercise increases the oxidative abilities of muscle tissue and trains the body to draw on its stores of fat for energy. Studies also show a happy additional benefit of exercise: Regular exercise increases the overall body metabolism for up to 24 hours after a workout. In other words, even when you are not working out, you are burning more calories than you would be if you had not exercised.

Will exercise that makes you perspire heavily help you lose weight?
You do not "sweat off" fat. Extremely vigorous exercise can make you sweat off three quarts of fluid hourly, but once you replace that fluid, as you should after a workout, you will regain those six pounds.

Do athletes need special food for energy?
No. Athletes and nonathletes alike require a solid, well-balanced diet, but nothing else. Athletes and their coaches used to believe that a high-protein diet was good for athletic performance, but that is not

true. In fact, what athletes need for endurance — as everyone does — is carbohydrates. If your carbohydrate intake is insufficient, you may notice that you suffer from fatigue, possibly even chronic fatigue. But no special diet is required for active people. See pages 125-127 for the place of carbohydrates in a balanced diet.

Is it safe to exercise during pregnancy?

You ought to check with your physician, but, as a general rule, you can exercise regularly during a normal pregnancy. Some studies indicate that women who exercise during pregnancy have fewer post-delivery complications than sedentary women. Walking, cycling, running and swimming are usually recommended for pregnant women.

Are some people better suited for exercise than others?

To be sure, everyone is unique. Age and sex affect performance in some exercises, and some people have a hereditary predisposition to do certain activities well. Human skeletal muscles are comprised of two basic types of muscle fibers: slow-twitch and fast-twitch. Slow-twitch fibers are better able to use oxygen for the production of energy. Although they do not have great strength, they are fatigue-resistant. Fast-twitch fibers, on the other hand, can contract quickly and forcefully. They provide strength, though they tire rapidly.

Some people are born with a greater-than-average proportion of one kind of muscle fiber. An elite marathon runner, for example, may have 80 to 90 percent slow-twitch muscle fibers, whereas a sprinter may have 70 percent fast-twitch fibers. No amount of training will change this distribution of fibers or enable either athlete to excel at the other's special event.

Nonetheless, endurance improves with training, no matter who you are. With a good aerobic exercise program, you may see your own VO$_2$max rise by at least 10 to 20 percent. Physiologists have reported improvements as high as 75 percent in some individuals.

Are there some exercises that wear down the body?

Many people believe that exercise will eventually take its toll on overused joints. Actually, there is no evidence that this is so. In fact, recent studies show that those who exercise regularly are less likely to develop degenerative joint disease than those who do not. Rather than breaking down bones and joints, running and other aerobic exercises add mass and strength to bones.

On the other hand, exercises can cause injuries — especially if the exercises are overdone, done incorrectly or done too frequently. About 40 percent of participants in aerobic movement classes, for instance, suffer from injuries severe enough for them to curtail taking classes or seek professional medical care. The majority of the injuries from aerobic dance, as from running, are stress, or overuse, injuries. Rest is the usual treatment for stress injuries.

O*nce considered the limit of human abilities, the 26.2-mile marathon foot race is now a popular event run not only by Olympic-level athletes, but by many others. Marathon participants frequently include wheelchair entrants, cardiac patients and the elderly. Between 500,000 and 700,000 Americans have completed the distance.*

Is exercising in a big city harmful to the lungs?

Many fitness enthusiasts are concerned with the effects of environmental pollution. Exposure to high concentrations of ozone, like those often found in the Los Angeles area, can cause chest tightness, headache, nausea, throat irritation and burning eyes. One study revealed that running for half an hour in heavy New York City traffic is the equivalent of smoking one half to one pack of cigarettes. High levels of carbon monoxide from automobile exhaust can extend as far as 60 feet from roadways. If you must exercise near heavily trafficked areas, it is best to work out in the early morning or late evening and stay at least 60 to 75 feet away from the traffic. Large parks with ample vegetation and wooded areas provide environmentally safe havens for anyone who exercises.

If you stop exercising, will you lose all of the benefits you have worked for?

No matter how long you have been exercising, you must continue your exercise program in order to maintain the training benefits, although you can take a couple of weeks off without losing all you have gained. In a study of athletes who had maintained their exercise programs for 10 years or more and then stopped training, researchers found that their aerobic capacities diminished gradually. After about 12 weeks, the athletes' maximal stroke volume — the amount of blood the heart can pump with one beat — was about the same as that of sedentary control subjects. Nevertheless, the athletes were able to return to their original aerobic capacities with only eight weeks of retraining.

Isn't it too late to get fit after age 55 or 60?

Virtually anyone, regardless of age or physical condition, can benefit from exercise. In one study, men aged 63 and older were found to increase their VO_2max as much as 49 percent through training.

Can exercise actually reverse "the aging process"?

Certainly not. However, physiologists have been struck by the similarities between the effects of sedentary living and aging, so much so that many scientists have concluded that many of the "normal symptoms of aging" may be in part symptoms of inactivity. Such effects include changes in the cardiovascular and respiratory system, cholesterol levels, bone mineral mass, joint flexibility, bowel function, immune system function, sleep patterns, sensory abilities and intellectual capacity. By age 60, for example, blood flow to the arms and the legs is 30 to 60 percent slower and muscle power is 10 to 30 percent less than what it was at age 25. By age 70, the metabolic rate has declined by 10 percent from that of a 25-year-old, the speed at which nerve messages travel has dropped 10 to 15 percent, flexibility has declined 20 to 30 percent, and bone mass has decreased by 15 to 30 percent. Each of these progressive dysfunctions can be postponed to some extent with regular aerobic exercise.

After 30 years of age, most people lose eight to 10 percent of their VO$_2$max every decade. By engaging in an aerobic conditioning program, however, elderly people can not only halt the decline in their aerobic power, but may actually raise their level of aerobic endurance to that of the average sedentary person 25 to 45 years their junior. One such person is Mavis Lindgren, a marathon record holder for women above the age of 65, who at age 78 recorded a VO$_2$max nearly equal to that of the average sedentary college-age woman.

Does exercise prevent heart attacks?

Heart disease is the nation's number one killer, striking more than a million people a year and killing almost half of them. More people die from heart ailments than from any other disease, including all forms of cancer. Epidemiological evidence suggesting that exercise and physical activity reduce the risk of heart disease was first put forward in 1953. Since then, numerous studies have noted a relationship between physical activity and protection from cardiovascular disease. Perhaps the most comprehensive series of studies on exercise and health is Dr. Ralph S. Paffenbarger's research on nearly 17,000 Harvard alumni. According to his studies, men who used up more than 2,000 calories a week in exercise had a 39 percent lower risk of heart attack than those who exercised less.

Exercise also appears to reduce the incidence of hypertension, sometimes called "the silent killer." Hypertension, or high blood pressure, has been linked to kidney failure, stroke and heart attack. In their studies of Harvard alumni, Dr. Paffenbarger and his associates found that men who did not engage in regular, vigorous exercise were at a 35 percent greater risk of developing hypertension at some time in their lives than those who did.

Aerobic exercise may also help raise the level of a protective cholesterol-carrying protein in the blood. This protein, called high-density lipoprotein (or HDL cholesterol), mops up excess low-density lipoprotein (or LDL cholesterol) in the blood and brings it back to the liver for reprocessing. It is LDL cholesterol that clogs up the blood vessels and causes heart attacks and strokes.

If exercise is good for you, why do people sometimes die during a workout?

On a muggy afternoon in July 1984, Jim Fixx, author of the best-selling *The Complete Book of Running* and a man who regularly jogged 10 miles a day, died suddenly of a heart attack while running.

An autopsy revealed that Fixx, 52 years old, had arteriosclerosis, which severely restricted blood flow to his heart muscle. The arteriosclerosis probably resulted from a number of factors, including an inherited predisposition to coronary artery disease and a decade or more of heavy cigarette smoking (he quit 15 years before he died), job stress and obesity. Although Fixx successfully eliminated most of these risk factors — and quite possibly prolonged his life — the damage to

A *re people who habitually exercise too tired for sex? To the contrary, one authoritative study found that married couples who engage in an exercise program report an increase in both the frequency and the quality of their sex.*

Exercise and Longevity Chart

Percent reduction in risk of death

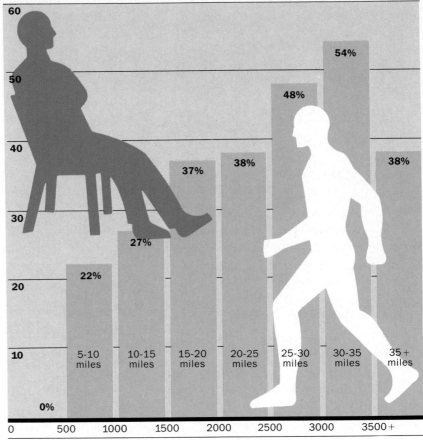

The more you exercise, the more likely you are to outlive your sedentary peers, according to a major study of nearly 17,000 Harvard alumni conducted by Dr. Ralph S. Paffenbarger and his associates. Men whose exercise used up fewer than 500 calories a week formed the group with the highest death rate, a rate the researchers defined as a 100 percent risk of death. Compared with this group, men who expended 500 to 1,000 calories a week — the rough equivalent of walking five to 10 miles — had a 22 percent lower risk of death. This relative improvement in longevity rose to 54 percent as calories expended increased to 3,500 a week — roughly, five to 10 hours of intense exercise. Among men who exercised more than that, however, the reduction in the risk of death went down slightly, to 38 percent, possibly because of hazards associated with demanding sports.

Activity in calories burned per week

his heart remained. Fixx had apparently refused to have a complete medical exam or take a stress test, which probably would have revealed the extent of the disease. Endurance athletes, especially those with multiple risk factors, should have regular checkups.

Since half a million Americans die of heart attacks each year, chance alone dictates that some of these deaths will occur during or immediately after exercise; however, exercise-related deaths are rare. One study of active males between the ages of 30 and 64 calculated that the risk of their dropping dead while running was 1 in 7,620. A study of 2,606 sudden deaths in Finland found that 22 were associated with exercise — 16 with skiing, two with jogging and four with other activities. The incidence of sudden death among Finnish sauna bathers, incidentally, was almost three times that of the exercisers.

Is exercise completely safe?
No. Even though dropping dead during exercise is rare, exercise does

carry some short-term risk of sudden death. Sedentary men greatly increase their chances of heart attack by engaging sporadically in vigorous activities (like shoveling snow). Even physically active people have a slightly higher risk of dying from a heart attack during an exercise session, although their overall risk of sudden death is 60 percent less than that of sedentary men. In other words, if you want to increase your chances of living through the next hour, go lie down and take it easy. If you want to have the best chance of living through the next 10 years or so, start an aerobic exercise program.

Is it true that exercise reduces the risk of cancer?

A study of 2,950 colon cancer cases in Los Angeles County found that the risk of colon cancer in men diminished as the level of physical activity increased. And a study conducted at Harvard University determined that women who were athletic in college and who continued an active life after graduation were less likely to develop cancers of the breast and reproductive system than were their less active female classmates. Statistically, sedentary women are three times as likely to develop reproductive system cancers and about twice as likely to develop breast cancers as active women.

Will exercise help you live longer?

The old joke that exercise will not make you live longer, only make your life seem longer, has finally been put to rest by Dr. Paffenbarger's study of Harvard alumni. The results indicate that men who exercise regularly can expect to add, on average, about two years to their lives. Two years may not sound like much at first. But that is an increase in life expectancy on the magnitude of a tremendous medical breakthrough — a cure for cancer.

To achieve a two-year increase in life expectancy, you must expend at least 2,000 calories a week in vigorous physical activity. Most people who engage in regular aerobic exercise and who are relatively active on a daily basis (for example, routinely climbing stairs and walking instead of driving) should easily expend 2,000 calories or more a week. For men between the ages of 35 and 54 who exercise regularly, this represents 2.5 additional hours of life for every one hour spent exercising.

Dr. Paffenbarger's study seems to indicate that there is a point of diminishing returns, however. The benefits remain constant when your exercise-related caloric expenditure exceeds 3,500 weekly, while the hazards of exercise (sudden death and accidents among them) increase, although only slightly.

What is the best possible exercise?

Any vigorous activity that uses the large skeletal muscles and can be maintained continuously for at least 20 minutes is perfectly acceptable. To begin designing the best exercise program for yourself, turn to the next page.

How to Design Your Own Program

Fitness is not merely a matter of working out or eating right. It is, rather, the cumulative effect of our style of living. Most of us would like to have a good idea of just how fit we are, and answering a few simple questions is all it takes. The questions and answers at right provide a starting point to assess your level of fitness — and to get your bearings for an aerobic conditioning program.

How fit are you?

1 How many times a week do you exert yourself vigorously — enough to work up a sweat — for 20 minutes or more?

If your answer is less than twice weekly, you are probably not at the top of your form. To maintain a moderate level of fitness, you need to work up a sweat twice a week; to be at an optimum level, three times a week.

2 Are you physically active at your job?

If you spend most of your day walking, climbing stairs and lifting packages, you may already be fit. A study of London bus personnel found that the conductors, who spend their day standing and climbing the stairs to the upper level of the buses, have a considerably lower death rate from heart disease than the drivers, who sit all day. If your job keeps you seated most of the day, you would do well to exercise in your free time.

3 Do you watch your weight?

A bit of fat will not shorten your lifespan. But if you are obese, that extra weight places a burden on virtually all your organs, and especially on your heart. The only good way to lose excess pounds is to eat a balanced diet with a moderate calorie intake — and to do aerobic exercise.

4 Have you had your blood pressure checked?

Fitness offers benefits for everyone, but it is especially beneficial for people whose blood pressure is too high. Since high blood pressure places severe strains on the cardiovascular system, it is one of the leading causes of strokes and heart attacks. You should therefore have your blood pressure checked regularly and if it is too high, take steps to reduce it. Depending on what causes the condition, you may be able to lower your blood pressure through diet (reducing your consumption of salt, for example), medication, exercise or a combination of the three. In some cases, aerobic conditioning alone is enough to reduce your blood pressure to safer levels.

5 Are you generally content and positive in your outlook?

Recent studies have proved what folk wisdom has long taught: Stress and depression can lower the body's resistance to disease. And one of the best ways to alleviate stress and depression is aerobic exercise.

6 Do you take time out of each day to relax?

Whether it is aerobic exercise or sports, working in your garden, strolling through a park or playing with your children, adults need to play to stay at the peak of health. People who can relax and "tune out" have been found to suffer fewer illnesses — and may live longer. And then there is the effect of laughter, an especially human form of relaxation. According to the Laughter Project at the University of California at Santa Barbara, laughter can reduce stress as effectively as certain complex biofeedback training programs can. And, unlike the biofeedback technique, laughter needs no special equipment.

7 Are you doing anything to control your cholesterol levels?

Cholesterol deposits in the arteries lead to heart disease, the number one cause of death in the United States. Most people ought to cut down on eggs, fatty meat, whole milk and such saturated fats as butter and bacon fat, which produce cholesterol that accumulates on the walls of blood vessels and impairs or cuts off circulation. On the other hand, replacing these saturated fats with modest amounts of polyunsaturated fats (corn, soy and safflower oil) can decrease overall cholesterol levels, especially the level of LDL, a cholesterol-carrying protein implicated in the build-up of cholesterol in the blood vessels. Sources of fiber like apples, carrots, nuts, soybeans and oatmeal also decrease blood cholesterol. In addition, most experts recommend aerobic exercise at least three times a week.

8 When you work out, do you monitor yourself to avoid overexertion?

Though a regular exercise program is crucial to your health, overdoing it will wear down your body, not build up your cardiovascular fitness. And if you exert yourself to the point that your heartbeat hits its maximum rate, you will quickly exhaust yourself. Use the chart on target heart rate *(page 24)* to monitor your aerobic workout.

How hungry are you?

People often say there is no point in exercising to lose weight because exercise just makes them hungry. Several studies have shown, however, that exercise actually decreases appetite. In one study, obese women participated in a moderate exercise program for eight weeks. Even though there were no limits on their caloric intake, the women ate less and lost an average of about 15 pounds each.

The Step Test

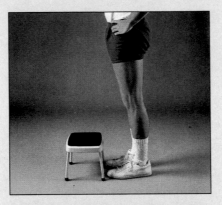

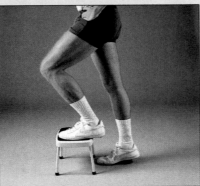

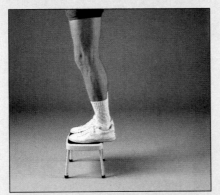

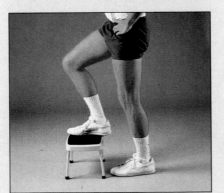

The three-minute step test, illustrated at left, is a simple measurement of aerobic fitness that you can conduct at home. It indicates your heart's ability to recover from mild exertion: A quick recovery is considered by physiologists to be a sign of fitness.

Although it is not meant to diagnose heart trouble or illness, the test is a useful tool for determining your present level of fitness and the intensity at which you should start exercising. By taking the test at least once a month, you can see how well your heart is adapting to exercise. The test is quite safe. However, people who have any sign of heart trouble, or who are over 35 years old and have not exercised for a year or more, should consult a physician before performing the test.

Taking the test

1. Find or construct a step or stool eight inches high.

2. Practice performing the step test so that you complete two up-up-down-down cycles in five seconds, as shown at left. A partner can be helpful in counting off the time. Rest a few minutes before the actual test.

3. Step up and down for exactly three minutes. After stopping, sit down, rest for 30 seconds and find your pulse. Then count your pulse for another 30 seconds. Compare the result with the chart at right.

Stand in front of an eight-inch step and step up and down in the sequence at left. Do two cycles every five seconds for three minutes, rest for 30 seconds and take your pulse.

STEP TEST RESULTS

☐ ☐ ☐ ☐ ☐ ☐ ☐ ☐ ☐ ☐ ☐ ☐

Enter your step test result in the first box above. Then find your fitness rating in the table below, which shows standard pulse counts according to sex, age and fitness level. After you start exercising, take the step test monthly and use the remaining boxes to track your improvement. (Read the suggestion at right for exercise in your classification.)

Classification	Age			
	20-29	30-39	40-49	50 & older
Men	**Number of beats**			
Excellent	34-36	35-38	37-39	37-40
Good	37-40	39-41	40-42	41-43
Average	41-42	42-43	43-44	44-45
Fair	43-47	44-47	45-49	46-49
Poor	48-59	48-59	50-60	50-62
Women	**Number of beats**			
Excellent	39-42	39-42	41-43	41-44
Good	43-44	43-45	44-45	45-47
Average	45-46	46-47	46-47	48-49
Fair	47-52	48-53	48-54	50-55
Poor	53-66	54-66	55-67	56-66

What to do next

Poor or Fair

You need an aerobic exercise program. Find the exercise that best fits your lifestyle and start at a beginning level, as shown on page 27.

Average

You need to exercise more regularly. Make sure you exercise for at least 20 minutes a day three times a week.

Good

You are in good shape, but there is still room for improvement. Increase the intensity or duration of your aerobic workouts.

Excellent

Keep doing what you are doing.

Taking Your Pulse

The best spot to measure your pulse is at the radial artery in your wrist. Although the pulse from the carotid artery in your neck is often easier to locate, studies show that this pulse can yield an inaccurate reading. Pressing the area around the carotid artery may decrease your heart rate, probably because the pressure from your fingers acts on nerves affecting cardiovascular activity, dropping it by more than 15 beats per minute.

Find your pulse using the sensitive tips of your index and middle fingers, as shown here. First feel for the wristbone at the base of the thumb, then move your fingertips toward your wrist. You will feel your pulse in a pocket of flesh.

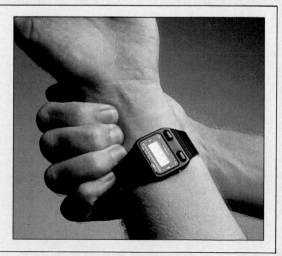

How Exercises Compare

EXERCISE	ADVANTAGES	DISADVANTAGES	CALORIES PER 1/2 HR.*
WALKING AND RACE WALKING	Good for anyone beginning an exercise program; very low injury rate; primarily conditions leg muscles, though race walking also works upper body; can be done anytime, anywhere; equipment: good shoes.	Heart rate is not elevated as easily as with some other exercises; therefore it may take longer to produce the same benefits.	2.5 mph: 105 4.5 mph: 200 6 mph:　370
AEROBIC MOVEMENT	Good exercise that can be done in classes or at home; can work all body parts; music adds to enjoyment; equipment: shoes designed for aerobics and a mat or suitable floor.	Relatively high injury rate in lower leg and foot; with low-impact aerobics, it is harder to raise heart rate.	light:　　120 moderate: 200 vigorous: 300
RUNNING	Very efficient conditioner: less time needed to achieve the same effects as walking; can be done anywhere; running clubs and competitions widely available for incentive; equipment: good running shoes.	Too strenuous for some people, and stress injuries are common.	5.5 mph: 320 6 mph:　350 7.5 mph: 430 10 mph: 550
CYCLING	Conditions lower body if done strenuously; low stress-injury rate; scenery and speed part of its appeal; can be done indoors on an exercise bike.	Expensive equipment: a bicycle with at least 10 gears, a safety helmet; injuries due to collision can occur; requires access to a long stretch of well-paved road.	5.5 mph: 130 10 mph:　220 13 mph:　320
SWIMMING	Excellent conditioner for whole body, particularly upper body, when done strenuously; extremely low injury rate; can be done by people with orthopedic injuries or disabilities.	Convenient access to a pool or other water necessary; can seem solitary; potential for eye and ear ailments.	25 yds/min: 180 40 yds/min: 260 50 yds/min: 375
CROSS–COUNTRY SKIING	Total body conditioner; low-impact activity with low injury rate; as scenic as downhill skiing, but more accessible.	Expensive equipment; requires convenient access to snowy trails; not a year-round option for most.	light:　　200 vigorous: 410+
ROWING	Superb exercise for the whole body, particularly the back; low impact and low injury rate; best on water, though indoor rowing machines provide similar fitness benefits.	Expensive equipment; a calm lake or river is a prerequisite.	light:　　200 vigorous: 420

*Approximate caloric expenditure for a person weighing 150 lbs. Add 10 percent for every 15 lbs. over this weight and subtract 10 percent for every 15 lbs. under.

Choosing an Exercise

A minimum requirement for aerobic exercise is that it provide continuous exertion to work the heart. Any of the activities in the chart at left can do this. They are also exercises you can take up at any age and practice for a lifetime.

Is one better than another? Theoretically, the most effective exercise is the one that promotes the highest VO_2max — the rating that indicates how efficiently your system can process oxygen for energy. Unless you are a competitive athlete training at high intensity, though, your heart does not care what kind of exercise you choose: You can work out at the same intensity whether you cycle, swim, row or run. But your mind does care. Studies show that people tend to stick with exercises that are accessible to them and the most enjoyable to perform. It is senseless to embark on a program at a health club that is distant from your home or office; despite your sincere intentions, chances are you will drop out.

If you live near a YMCA, however, and you enjoy swimming, then you should seriously consider beginning a swimming program. If you live near a park or in the country, then running, walking or cycling may be your best choice. If there is snow, you can take up cross-country skiing several months a year.

You should also consider the additional nonaerobic benefits an exercise offers, along with the types of injuries that are possible. Swimming, cross-country skiing and rowing have lower injury rates than aerobic movement, running or cycling, but the latter are usually more accessible. You have to take your own physical condition into account, too. If you have back trouble, for example, running may aggravate it. A better choice would be cycling, which jars the back less. The following chapters cover in detail the benefits and potential stresses of each exercise, as well as the techniques and equipment for getting the most out of it.

As a way of enhancing overall fitness, you may eventually want to consider taking up two or more exercises, or "cross-training." As explained on page 26, cross-training can also lower your chance of injury and will give your program more variety. Studies show that variety is one of the keys to staying motivated.

Staying with it

For many people, the hardest part of an exercise program is not learning what to do or how to do it, but doing it regularly. Though it is difficult to predict who will drop out of any particular exercise program, half of the participants can be expected to drop out within six months to a year of starting a supervised program. Even people who would seem to have compelling reasons for sticking with it drop out. In one study of post-heart attack patients put on an exercise program, 71 percent of the participants, all of whom had been referred to the hospital by a physician, stopped during the first two years.

The most important step when starting a program is to set realistic, attainable goals. If you are out of shape, do not try to run several miles or swim 50 laps in the first week or two. You are also better off concentrating on time, not on distance. Researchers have found that runners who aim for 30 minutes during an exercise session are more likely to keep running than those who go for mileage.

Second, there is a correlation between the intensity of the exercise and the propensity to quit. Far too often, people think that pushing themselves to the limit will accomplish the most. But unless you are training for competition, this is not true. The more intensely you exercise, the more quickly fatigue sets in — forcing you to stop short of your goal — and the rate of injury increases.

Third, you can heighten the pleasures of exercise with the following techniques:

- Find the right time. Some people discover that exercising early in the day supplies them with energy throughout the morning. For others, an after-work jog or swim releases the day's tensions. If your leisure time is short, you can walk or cycle to and from work.
- Monitor your progress. Keeping a chart of how often you exercise, and of the time that has elapsed or the distance you have covered, reinforces the feeling of personal achievement.
- Vary your exercise routine. Switch your walking routes for a change of scenery; swim in a lake instead of a pool; cover different types of terrain when cycling or cross-country skiing; instead of running continuously, intersperse the run with brief intervals of skiing, jumping, and running up and down stairs.
- Get the support of others. Social support, especially from family members, has been consistently linked with staying on an exercise program. In one study, people with spouses who actively supported their exercise regimen were twice as likely to keep going as those whose spouses were nonsupportive. And people who exercise in a group, researchers have found, are less likely to quit than those who exercise alone.
- Finally, do not worry if you miss a session or two, or if you do not consistently meet the time or distance goals you have set for yourself. The point is to not let lapses become a habit.

Your Target Heart Rate

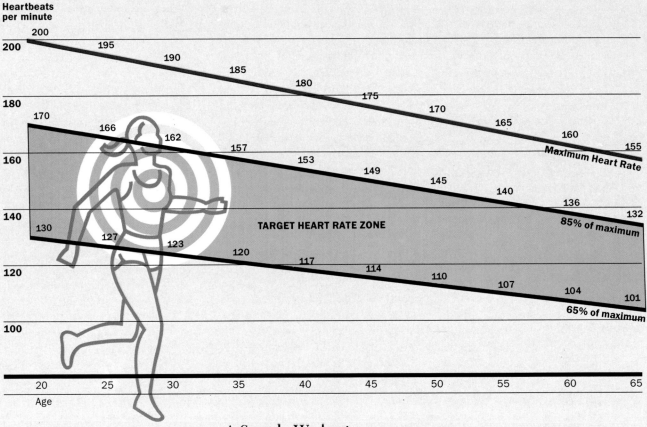

Heartbeats per minute

200
195
190
185
180
175
170
165
160
155

Maximum Heart Rate

170
166
162
157
153
149
145
140
136
132

85% of maximum

130
127
123
120
117
114
110
107
104
101

65% of maximum

TARGET HEART RATE ZONE

200
180
160
140
120
100

20 25 30 35 40 45 50 55 60 65

Age

A Sample Workout

To determine your target heart rate, find your age along the bottom of the chart above. Trace a line straight up to the lower edge of the shaded area; that pulse rate is the lower limit of your target heart rate. Continue the line to the top of the shaded area; that pulse rate is the upper limit of your target heart rate. Begin a workout with a five-minute warm-up that starts your heart climbing gradually toward its target zone, as shown at right. During training sessions, your heart rate should stay within that zone for at least 20 minutes, then descend slowly to its resting rate during the five-minute cool-down.

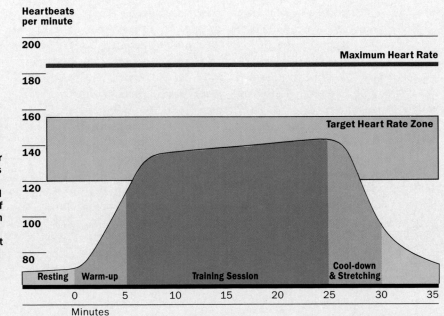

Heartbeats per minute

Maximum Heart Rate

Target Heart Rate Zone

200
180
160
140
120
100
80

Resting Warm-up Training Session Cool-down & Stretching

0 5 10 15 20 25 30 35

Minutes

24

Pacing your workout

The most important consideration when exercising is how hard to push yourself. If you exercise at too low an intensity, you will not achieve a training effect. If you push too vigorously, you will become fatigued. Fortunately, you need only one tool to guide you — your heart rate. Researchers have determined that most people can exercise safely and effectively when their heart rate increases to between 65 and 85 percent of their maximum heart rate (the upper limit of your heart's pumping ability). This 65-to-85-percent range is your target heart rate. Exercising below this range may make your progress frustratingly slow, while exceeding it can quickly cause exhaustion and possibly lead to stress injury.

Maximum heart rate decreases with age; therefore, you need to take your age into account when determining your target heart rate. You can use the chart on the opposite page to compute it. Physiologists have also devised this formula:
1) subtract your age from 220 (your theoretical maximum heart rate);
2) multiply that figure by .65 and also by .85. While you exercise, your heart rate per minute should remain between those two figures.

Studies indicate that exercising at the upper limit of your target heart rate is most effective. But exercising at the lower limit, which lessens the chance of strain or injury, is certainly intense enough to produce a training effect. At this lower heart rate, you should be able to carry on a conversation during a workout.

Check your heart rate when you exercise by pausing to take your pulse from the radial artery in your wrist.

Count it for 10 seconds and multiply the figure by six. If you find you are exercising below your target heart rate and are feeling no discomfort, you should gradually increase the intensity of your workout. Check your pulse frequently — about every five minutes. After you have been exercising regularly for a few weeks, you will learn to judge when you are in the target zone, so that you need on ly take your pulse once or twice during a workout.

The workout itself should consist of three phases: the warm-up, the training phase and the cool-down. The warm-up and cool-down, which are explained in detail on pages 28-29, are crucial for easing your heart into and out of your target zone. For the training phase, you must increase your pace to lift your heart into its target zone and keep it there for at least 20 minutes.

How long and how often you should work out depends on your present condition and your goals, as explained on pages 26-27. In general, though, when you begin an exercise program, you should stay toward the lower end of your target heart rate zone during the training phase of your workout. Once you can exercise comfortably at that level, you can gradually increase your intensity to the 75-to-85-percent range.

As you become more fit, you will need to exercise more vigorously to raise your heart rate. Yet the added exertion will not feel any more strenuous: This energy dividend is the most basic reward of aerobic conditioning. It is the result — and the proof — of having strengthened your heart and the muscles you have been using to exercise it.

Heart Rate Conversion Table

10-second count	Heartbeats per minute	
32	192	
31	186	
30	180	
29	174	
28	168	
27	162	
26	156	85%
25	150	
24	144	
23	138	
22	132	
21	126	
20	120	65%
19	114	
18	108	
17	102	
16	96	
15	90	
14	84	
13	78	
12	72	
11	66	
10	60	
9	54	
8	48	

Target heart rate for a 35-year-old

When you exercise, you should calculate your heart rate by counting your pulse for 10 seconds. (If you stop to take your pulse for a full minute, it will already have slowed down by the time 60 seconds have elapsed.) Once you know your target heart rate *(opposite page)*, locate it in the column at right, then find the corresponding 10-second pulse counts. The numbers at the upper and lower limit are the ones you need to remember to monitor your workout. A 35-year-old man, for example, should be sure that his pulse count always falls between 20 and 26.

Setting Your Level

Once you have chosen an exercise, you can decide how to put it to work for you over the long run. The guidelines on the opposite page, which offer three levels of aerobic exercise, allow you to design a program to suit your physical condition and weekly schedule. Three key factors shape a program at each level: the frequency of exercise sessions, their duration and their intensity (as measured by your target heart rate).

The level you set depends upon your physical condition, your goals and your schedule. If you exercise primarily to improve cardiovascular fitness, you will find the optimum level — which requires workouts three or four days a week — to be the most suitable. This level offers the greatest amount of benefit without requiring major changes in your schedule. If you want first and foremost to lose weight, however, you may want to exercise five times a week in order to expend more calories. (To lose weight efficiently, of course, you must also control your diet.) To give your heart maximum pumping ability or to train for competition in endurance events calls for an even greater investment of time. At this higher level, the chances of injury are also greater.

Whatever your goals, above all give yourself time to progress. Studies show that the most common mistake is beginning an exercise program too aggressively. People try to do too much too soon; as a result, they tire quickly, become discouraged and increase their chances of getting injured. Even if you consider yourself in good condition and perform well on the step test (pages 20-21), start any new exercise slowly. You can greatly reduce the risk of injury by following these guidelines:

- Work through the beginning level first.
- Increase the training phase of your workouts by no more than 10 percent a week.
- After you have met the demands of a certain level, stick with it for eight to 10 weeks before moving up to the next level.

Cross-Training

The most practical and effective way to achieve aerobic fitness is to use one exercise. You will rapidly build up your ability to sustain it — and that is the whole point of aerobic exercise. But staying with one activity has its limitations: It can be monotonous, and it usually develops some muscles while leaving others undeveloped. You can expand the challenge and the benefits of a fitness program by cross-training, or training in more than one activity.

The most ardent practitioners of cross-training are triathletes, who train and compete in running, swimming and cycling. They maintain that you can best condition your entire body and most of your muscle groups by working out regularly in these three activities. But you do not have to do all three activities, or those particular three. More practically, you can cross-train by doing two exercises — running and swimming, for example — on alternate days. Or you can switch over on a seasonal basis — for example, cross-country skiing in the winter and cycling or running the rest of the year.

The most immediate benefit of cross-training is the mental change of pace it provides, especially when you feel that you can barely force yourself to plod through one more workout. Another benefit is that you can maintain aerobic fitness year-round despite an injury or a change in season. Runners, for example, can take up swimming not only as a winter activity, but also to recover from running injuries that involve muscles different from those used for swimming.

Because different exercises condition different sets of muscles, cross-training will also give you a better physique. By combining swimming with activities like running or cycling, you can build your upper and lower body uniformly. Furthermore, this extensive muscle development reduces the chance of your getting injured while exercising. In endurance activities, many injuries are caused by muscle imbalance, which occurs when one muscle group becomes stronger than an opposing group. Running, for example, strengthens the hamstring muscles on the back of the thigh, but not the quadriceps in the front. By adding cycling, which does work the quadriceps, you can better balance the two muscle groups and lessen the chance of pulled muscles or knee injuries.

Less clear is the extent to which cross-training benefits your endurance. Physiologists have found that doing one type of exercise regularly and well does not enable you to take up a new exercise at the same intensity. The reason is that only conditioned muscles can take full advantage of the extra oxygen that the heart and lungs in a fit body are able to deliver. In one study, a group of men who trained on stationary bicycles for eight weeks improved their VO_2max by 7.8 percent. However, when the subjects were tested on a treadmill, their improvement was only 2.6 percent. In a similar test, conditioned swimmers who were put on a treadmill tired quickly.

Based on these findings, you should not expect cross-training to improve your performance substantially in any one activity. You can raise your endurance as a runner, for example, only by running. When you start a new exercise, do so gradually, regardless of your fitness level. If you are substituting one activity for another, taper off the old one as you build endurance in the new one. If you decide to cross-train frequently, alternate activities and increase your training time in each at the rate of 10 percent a week, just as you would with a single exercise.

Beginning level

◆ If you are out of shape or want to begin a new exercise, this is the level to start at. It will give you a solid aerobic base; less exercise than this may produce only minimal benefits. You should aim for three 30-minute workouts a week, each with a five-minute warm-up, a 20-minute training phase and a five-minute cool-down. The workouts should be spaced at least two days apart in order to allow your muscles to recover. In four to six weeks, you should see an increase in endurance and a drop in your resting heart rate — both indications that your heart is pumping more efficiently. If you modify your diet, you may begin to lose body fat as well. Because exercise typically produces an increase in muscle mass, your weight may not drop. But since muscle tissue is leaner than fat, you will look and feel trimmer.

Optimum level

◆ By reaching this level, you will derive all of the benefits that aerobic exercise offers. Not only will your resting heart rate continue to drop, but your percentage of fat tissue should decrease farther. In addition, your percentage of lean muscle may increase, and your level of HDL cholesterol should rise. (HDL is the "good" type of cholesterol: It clears "bad," artery-clogging cholesterol out of your system.) At this level, you will be doing the most you can to protect yourself from a heart attack (short of giving up cigarettes if you smoke).

The most methodical schedule at this level is four weekly workouts of 40 minutes each: a five-minute warm-up, a 30-minute training phase and a five-minute cool-down. But because variety is a key factor in sticking with an exercise program, you should feel free to vary your schedule. You could spread your workouts over five days, which allows you to shorten the training phase to 20 minutes on some days. Or you could train for 45 minutes on Monday, 30 minutes on Wednesday and 45 again on Friday. Changing the length of a workout also allows you to take different routes when exercising outdoors.

Competitive level

◆ Exercise at this level takes you beyond what is required for cardiovascular fitness. You will continue to experience an improvement in aerobic capacity, but the improvement will not be nearly so dramatic as when moving through the previous levels. And at this level there is also a substantial investment in time along with a significant rise in the chance of injury. Therefore, your goal is no longer simply to get fit: Most people training at this level do so to condition themselves for competition in their chosen exercise.

You can be flexible designing your regimen. For example, you could work out in 40-minute training sessions six days a week, 48-minute sessions five days a week, or alternate 30-, 40- and 50-minute training sessions for six days of the week. A good way to avoid stress injuries and to stay fresh is to rest one day each week. To sustain your motivation, you can also alternate "hard" and "easy" workouts, a training technique used by most competitive athletes. On days when short workouts are scheduled, exercise at a relatively high intensity, close to the pace you would reach in competition. On days when your workout is 50 minutes, exercise at an easier pace, near the low end of your target heart rate zone.

Warm-Ups and Cool-Downs

Because the aerobic benefits and the exhilaration of doing an exercise come from pushing yourself, you may be tempted to skip warming up and cooling down. But regardless of how fit you are, both phases are vital for easing the body into and out of exercise. They reduce the muscle stiffness that can develop, they protect you from injuries, and they make the exercise itself more enjoyable.

A proper warm-up results in muscles that are more pliable, since loose, flexible muscles are less likely to be strained or pulled than tight ones. Realizing this, many people begin a workout by stretching. However, studies show that stretching cold muscles is not the right way to warm them up: You do not get as much benefit stretching a cold muscle as stretching a warmed-up muscle, and you might even hurt it. Nor does wearing a sweat suit help muscles warm up; all too often, in fact, wearing heavy sweat clothes simply interferes with the body's ability to cool itself.

The best way to warm up is to exercise at a light pace for five to six minutes, or until you begin to perspire. You can walk, jog or use another endurance activity. Warming up in this manner increases blood flow to muscles and tendons, raising their temperature, which increases their flexibility. A warm-up also prepares your heart to meet the muscles' increased demand for blood. In one study, 70 percent of the healthy males who took stress tests experienced abnormal heartbeats during exercise if they did not warm up beforehand. Warming up, however, eliminated the irregularities.

After you complete the training phase of your workout, cool down by slowing down. Physiologists have observed that stopping exercise abruptly can cause a sudden drop in blood pressure, potentially stressing the heart. You can lessen this stress by performing your exercise at a slower pace for five to 15 minutes until your breathing returns to normal. Ending your workout this way keeps blood flowing through working muscles, stabilizes blood pressure and lets your heart rate descend slowly and steadily.

You can enhance a warm-up and a cool-down with a moderate stretching routine. Although many people like to stretch before they start exercising, the benefit to muscles and tendons may be greater after you workout, when muscles have been warmed thoroughly.

The six exercises on the opposite page will stretch most of the muscle groups used in endurance activities. They are static stretches designed to loosen muscles gradually without straining them. Do not bounce or jerk when you perform them. Instead, slowly move into the position shown until you start to feel mild tension in the muscles. Hold that position for 10 to 30 seconds without fighting the muscles. Relax, then repeat the stretch several times, until the muscle feels pleasantly supple.

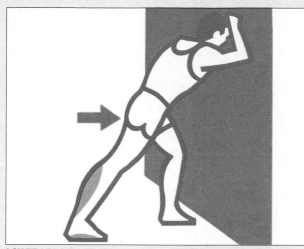

LOWER LEG STRETCH To loosen the calf muscles and connective tissues in the feet, lean against a wall and move your hips forward. Keep your rear foot flat and your knee straight. Repeat with the other leg.

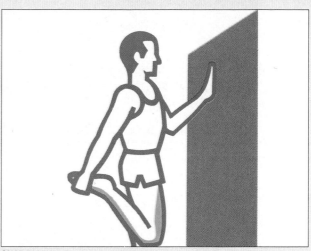

QUADRICEPS To stretch the large muscle in the front of your thigh, brace yourself against a wall and grasp one foot. Gently pull toward your buttocks, keeping your back straight. Repeat with the other leg.

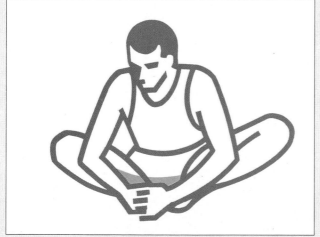

GROIN Sit on the ground with the soles of your feet together. Hold your toes and gently lean forward from the waist. You should feel the stretch not only in your groin, but in your inner thighs and lower back.

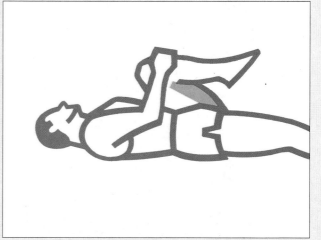

HAMSTRINGS AND LOWER BACK Lie on your back. Draw one knee toward your chest while keeping the other knee flat on the ground. Grasp your knee and gently pull it a bit farther. Repeat with the other leg.

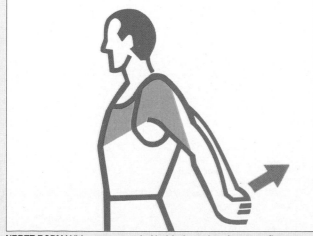

UPPER BODY With arms extended behind you, interlace your fingers and push up and back. Keep your chest out and your head erect. The stretch should flow down from your shoulders to your upper arms and chest.

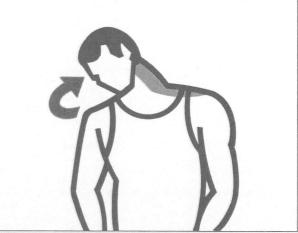

NECK Drop your head back and look straight up. Slowly roll your head to the left, then to the right. Repeat this movement, keeping your shoulders and back as straight as possible.

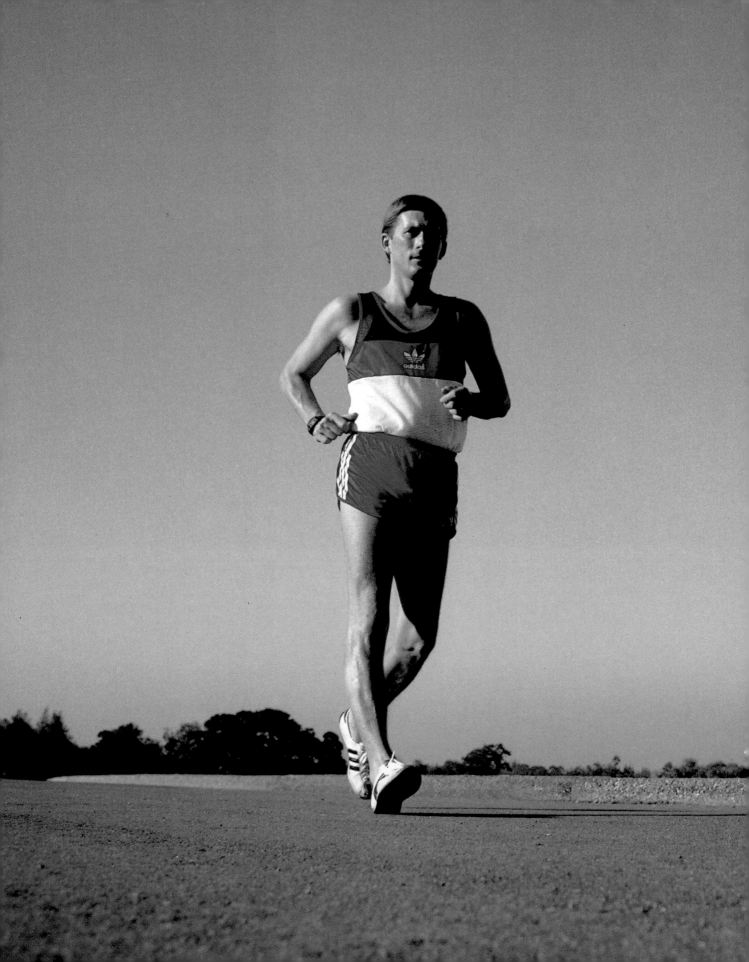

CHAPTER TWO

Walking

An activity for anyone — one that's even better than running

At first glance, walking may not seem like much of an exercise. After all, plenty of out-of-shape people walk. But, in fact, walking can provide virtually the same cardiovascular benefits as distance running. According to a large-scale survey of athletes, competitive walkers had about the same VO_2max values — the measurement of the body's ability to deliver oxygen to the working muscles — as ultramarathon runners and competitive cyclists. However, you can get many conditioning benefits without having to walk at a competitive level. In one study, a group of sedentary middle-aged subjects walked on a treadmill for 40 minutes four times a week. At the end of 20 weeks, their average VO_2max had increased by 28 percent and their heart rates during exercise had decreased anywhere from four to 17 beats per minute. The walkers also showed improved lung capacity and a drop in body fat.

In addition to its fitness benefits, walking is simple, safe and accessible to nearly everyone, all of which increase the chances of someone

31

sticking with a walking regimen. Among people who embark on exercise programs, walkers appear to have the lowest dropout rates. In one study, the dropout rate from a walking program was less than half that of most other activities.

It is true that walking at a casual pace will not provide much of a training effect for your cardiovascular system. Yet by using any of the three basic walking techniques, you can increase your cardiovascular workload and achieve as substantial a training effect with walking as with almost any other form of aerobic exercise.

Brisk walking (3-3.5 mph) is a slight extension of casual walking. People who can benefit especially from brisk walking are the elderly, those who are out of shape and want to ease slowly into an exercise program, and those recovering from surgery or a heart attack.

Striding (3.5-5.5 mph) is a further extension of simple walking, in which the legs extend boldly forward and the arms swing vigorously to intensify the effort. Many striders carry weights to increase their caloric expenditure and enhance the cardiovascular benefit of walking.

Race walking (5-9 mph) brings the entire body into action: It conditions the muscles of the shoulders, upper arms and trunk as well as the legs. As an aerobic exercise, race walking is not only superior to brisk walking and striding, it can equal running. Indeed, top race walkers can walk a mile in less than six minutes —faster than most people can run a mile.

In addition to effectively conditioning you, walking — compared with running and most other aerobic exercises — is a low-impact activity that rarely leads to injury. Walking uses a full heel-to-toe motion; the footstrike is at the back of the heel, and the pushoff is at the end of the big toe. This spreads the force of impact over the widest possible foot area, relieving any one spot of excessive stress. It also allows the foot to roll forward and provide momentum for the body. Runners, on the other hand, land more flat-footed with greater force and less roll, and then bounce into the air for a short period of time before striking the ground again. Walkers never lose contact with the ground: A walker's advancing foot lands before the rear foot leaves the ground. Except for blisters, which are primarily the result of ill-fitting shoes, exercise walkers are troubled only by occasional mild shin splints — tenderness between the ankle and the knee that can usually be treated with ice and a day or two of rest.

Because you can combine it with other activities, walking as an exercise is especially attractive to people who have difficulty carving time out of busy schedules for formal training sessions. You can walk around the block, walk to work, explore new neighborhoods or hike through the woods. Some walkers even work out in shopping malls.

Moreover, walking is an easy exercise to share. Most people find it less intimidating than any other form of exercise, and it should not be difficult to encourage friends and family to join you. Remember, though, that your choice of time, place and companions should allow

Walking Program Tips

◆ Start out by walking or striding at a pace that raises your heart rate into its target zone — unless your score on the step test was fair or poor, in which case you should walk at a pace that you find comfortable. Walk on alternate days, gradually increasing your pace until you can do one mile in about 15 minutes.

◆ Try walking at a regular cadence. For the first four or five weeks of your walking program, aim for a cadence of 90 to 120 steps per minute. (Going uphill, you will have to shorten your stride to keep the cadence regular.) As your fitness improves, your cadence must increase to keep your heart rate in its target zone.

◆ Moving faster is the best way to increase the workload of walking. However, many people will find it uncomfortable to walk faster than 140 or 150 steps per minute. Once you have reached that point, you can intensify your exercise effort in several ways. A hike along a rough but relatively level trail requires 50 percent more energy expenditure than walking on a paved road. You can also increase the exercise benefits by walking in hilly terrain or by loading yourself with extra weight, as explained on pages 36-37. Ascending a 15-degree slope, for example, requires nearly four times as much effort as walking on a level surface.

you to set a pace that keeps your heart rate in its target zone. Otherwise, you will not get a training effect.

The only equipment essential for walking is a good pair of shoes. Running shoes are suitable, though walking is so stress-free that you do not need the thick cushioning that running shoes provide. If you wish, you can buy shoes designed for exercise walking. These generally have thinner midsoles and lower heels than running shoes, and some — particularly those designed for race walking — have outsoles that wrap over the tip of the toe, facilitating the full heel-to-toe walking stride. However, almost any pair of flexible, supportive, well-fitted shoes will go a long way toward ensuring your comfort. Walking shoes made out of leather will require a break-in period to avoid blisters.

You should wear clothing that is appropriate to the climate. You can wear loose-fitting street clothes for brisk walking and striding, although a warm-up suit may be more comfortable. Race walking, because of its more dynamic movements, requires the same clothing as running. In colder weather, remember that 70 percent of the body heat you dissipate is lost through your head and hands. A wool cap and gloves will probably keep you reasonably warm.

In warm weather and under a direct sun, shield your head with a light cap that contains air pockets. Wear shorts, which allow greater freedom of movement than pants. It may be wise to rub petroleum jelly on the insides of your thighs — and under your arms if race walking — to prevent chafing.

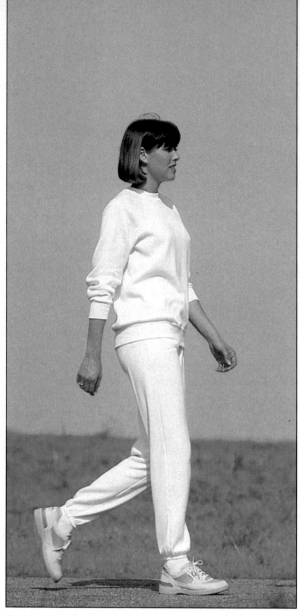

For good posture, keep your shoulders back and your head up.

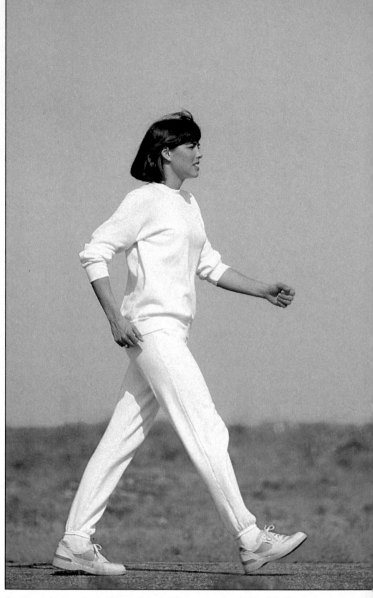

As you advance to brisk walking, let your arms swing freely.

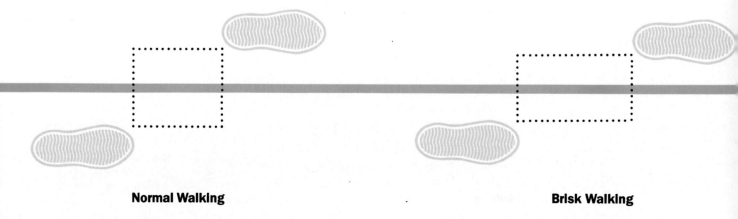

Normal Walking

Brisk Walking

From Walking To Striding

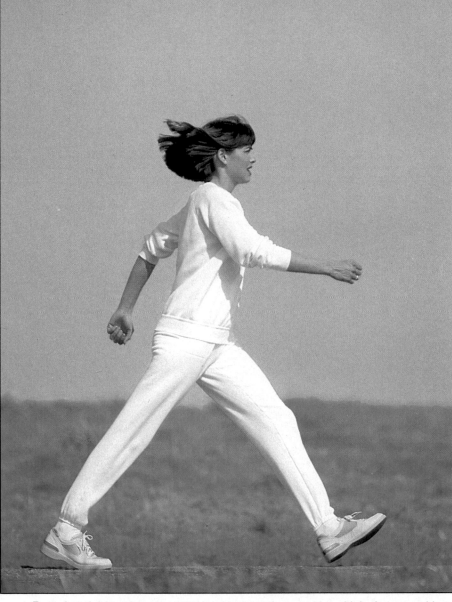

To go from brisk walking to striding, add energetic movement with both arms and legs.

Posture is the most fundamental aspect of good walking technique. Poor posture will shorten your stride, cause back pain or exhaust you before you have completed your workout. Be sure to walk erect. Do not bend over or look down at your feet. Leaning over while you walk will shorten your stride and can cause back pain and unnecessary fatigue. Keep your shoulders back, but not stiff, and breathe deeply. Your hands should be loose and unclenched; let them swing freely by your sides.

To move from walking to striding, you must swing your arms more vigorously and lengthen your stride. A full, strong arm swing is essential for balance, and it helps you breathe more regularly. As your pace picks up, your feet will land along a straighter line and with greater force. For maximum efficiency, swing your foot forward like a pendulum and plant the heel at about a 40-degree angle. Then roll forward to push off with your toe.

Striding

As you progress to striding *(left),* your stride lengthens and your feet land closer to an imaginary center line extending straight ahead of you.

Increasing the Effort

To increase the workload of brisk walking and striding, you can train on hills. This will not only raise your heart rate, but will burn extra calories as well. A 150-pound man, for instance, will expend about 285 calories in one hour of brisk walking. If he walks briskly up a moderate 10-degree incline, however, he can burn about 300 calories in just 25 minutes.

Most hills are not long enough to sustain an uphill walk of 25 minutes or more. One way to increase the effort is to carry weights — hand-held weights, backpacks or weighted belts. Researchers found that college-age men could improve their VO_2max by as much as 20 percent in four weeks by walking briskly (at about three miles per hour) for 30 minutes five times a week while carrying a backpack load weighing six to 12 pounds.

Carrying similar amounts of weight in the hands or strapped to the ankles is even more effective, according to a U.S. Army study. Most people, however, would find it uncomfortable to carry weights of more than six pounds. Hand weights of one to three pounds designed for walkers and joggers are available, though at least one study has shown that you must swing your arms vigorously to get any benefit from these lighter weights. Ankle weights are not recommended, since they may lead to injury.

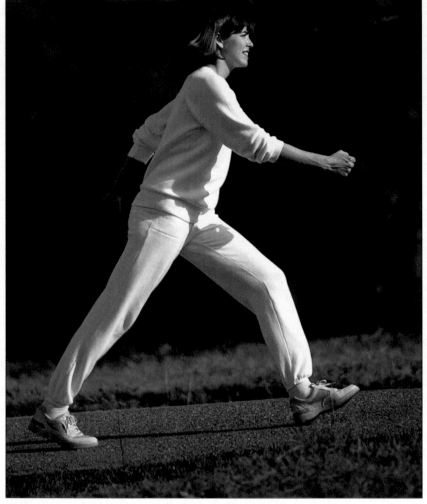

When walking up a hill, lean forward slightly and use a strong arm swing to keep moving powerfully. Continue to land on your heels, not flat-footed.

Walking with Hand Weights

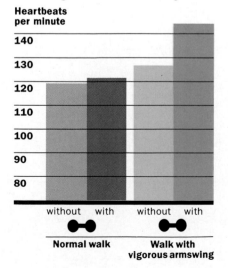

Heartbeats per minute

140
130
120
110
100
90
80

without   with
Normal walk

without   with
Walk with vigorous armswing

The chart at left, based on a study of college students, shows that carrying three-pound hand-held weights while walking barely increases the heart rate during exercise. Vigorous arm swinging while carrying the weights, however, raised the heart rate of subjects by an average of about 25 beats per minute.

To upgrade your walking with hand weights, swing your arms to at least chest level *(inset)*. A weighted belt increases the workload even further.

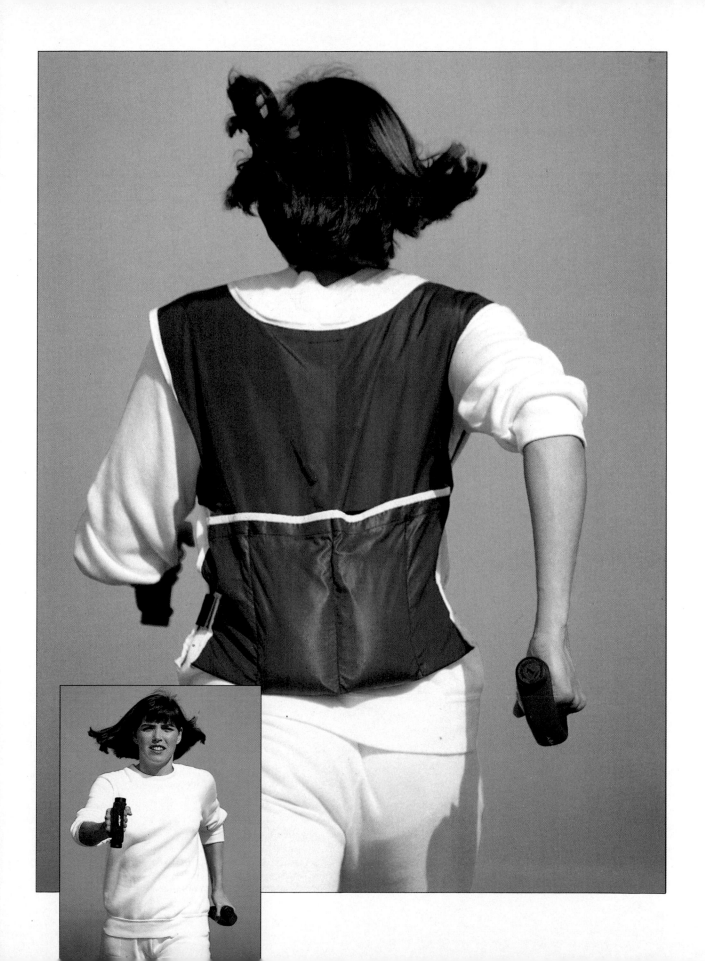

Race Walking

Race walking is not simply a more intense version of normal walking, but a unique form of motion, as different from normal walking as it is from running. With each stride, the race walker's upper and lower body move in coordinated opposition. The pelvis rotates dramatically, the arms pump forcefully with upper arm and forearm forming right angles. The legs work at a rapid cadence. Your workload increases over ordinary brisk walking for greater fitness benefits.

To race walk correctly, you should have a moment of double support, which means that your advancing foot must make contact with the ground before your rear foot leaves it. The supporting leg must be straight, with the knee locked when the body is upright. If you combine the right stride with the proper hip and arm movements *(pages 40-41)*, you will be moving as fast as many people run.

In addition to increasing your speed, race walking eliminates wasteful motions. During ordinary walking, your feet land on either side of an imaginary line running in the direction of travel; therefore, your body sways back and forth slightly as you transfer your weight from one foot to the other. Race walking directs your movement in a straight line — your feet should land almost directly in front of one another, as shown in the diagram opposite.

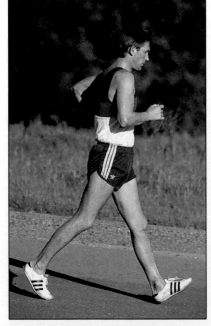

As you extend your advancing leg, straighten the knee as the heel hits the ground. Keep your arms bent at a right angle.

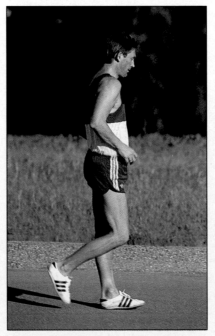

Lock your knee as soon as you land on your left foot. Push off and start to swing your right foot, keeping it low to the ground.

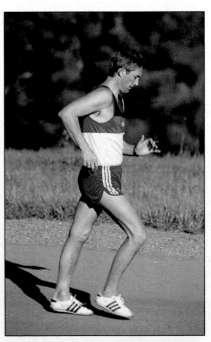

Continue to swing your right foot forward. Swing the left arm forward like a pendulum and pull your right arm back.

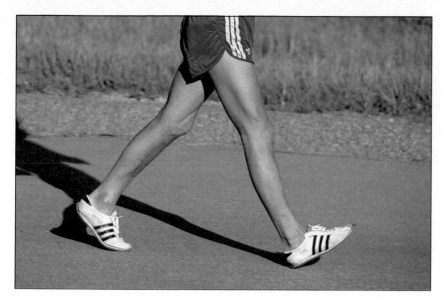

The most crucial moment of the race walking stride is the double-support phase, when both feet come into contact with the ground. Your rear foot should give a final push off with the toes as the heel of the forward foot strikes the ground. To maintain an efficient gait, the double-support phase should last only an instant. Top race walkers move through it in a few thousandths of a second.

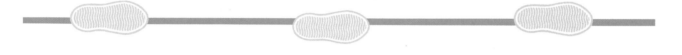

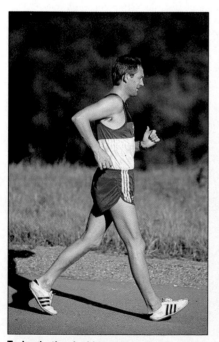

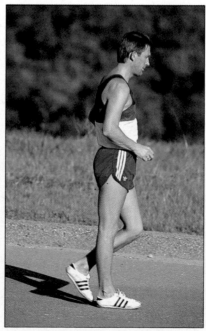

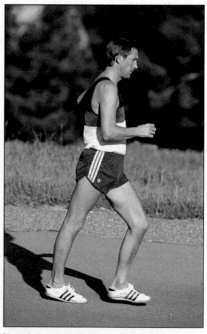

To begin the double-support phase, plant your right heel with the foot at a 40-degree angle. Swing your arms high.

As your body comes over the right leg, your arms and shoulders descend to their lowest position. Arms remain bent.

You then move into the next stride. Be sure to keep the right leg straightened as it pushes your body forward.

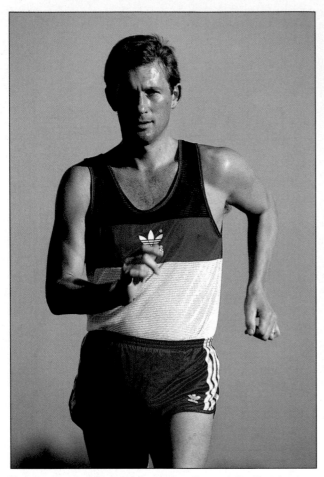 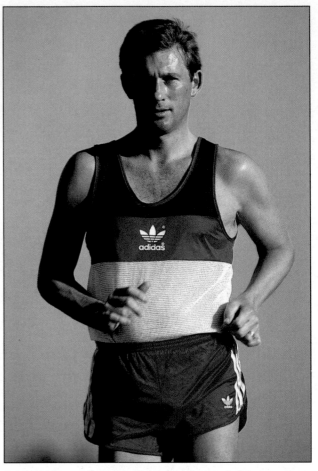

To help propel the left hip forward, pull your left elbow back while you swing your right arm forward.

At midstride, move your hands to waist level and align your upper body vertically over the supporting leg.

Hip and Arm Power

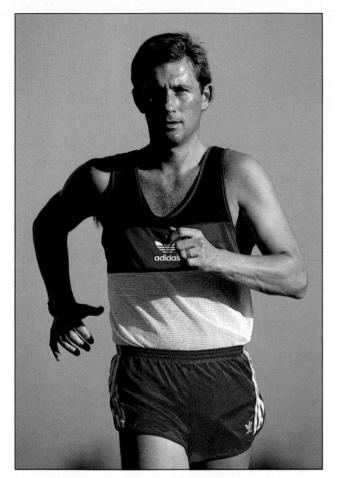

Even during the most vigorous portion of the stride, do not let your hands cross the midline of your chest.

Race walkers used to be called "wobblies" because of their unusual hip movements. In order to achieve the most efficient race-walking stride, the pelvis wobbles, or swivels. Because of this hip rotation, your center of gravity barely shifts up and down or from side to side, as it does during normal walking. You travel directly forward, almost gliding over the ground.

An added benefit of hip rotation is that it can increase the race walker's stride length by about 10 percent. A six-foot race walker, therefore, is capable of a stride length about seven inches longer than a six-footer who is walking fast but with a normal gait. And the race walker takes about 120 fewer steps per mile, a considerable saving in effort.

To develop hip rotation, concentrate on your arms, using them as pendulums to regulate the work of your hips and legs. Drive your arms into the movement of walking by pulling them backward with each step. These arm movements transmit forward force to your hips, helping you to move ahead. With each step, a slight forward rotation occurs at the shoulder as you swing one arm forward and pull the other arm back. These movements may feel unnatural at first, but, with practice, they should become second nature.

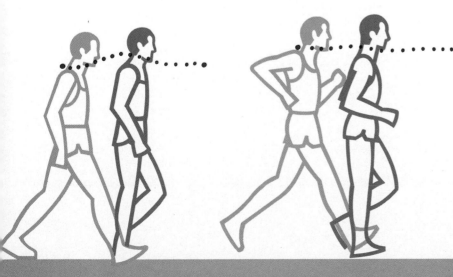

During normal brisk walking *(far left)*, your head and shoulders may move up and down about three inches with each stride. Race walking *(near left)* reduces this bobbing movement to less than an inch.

41

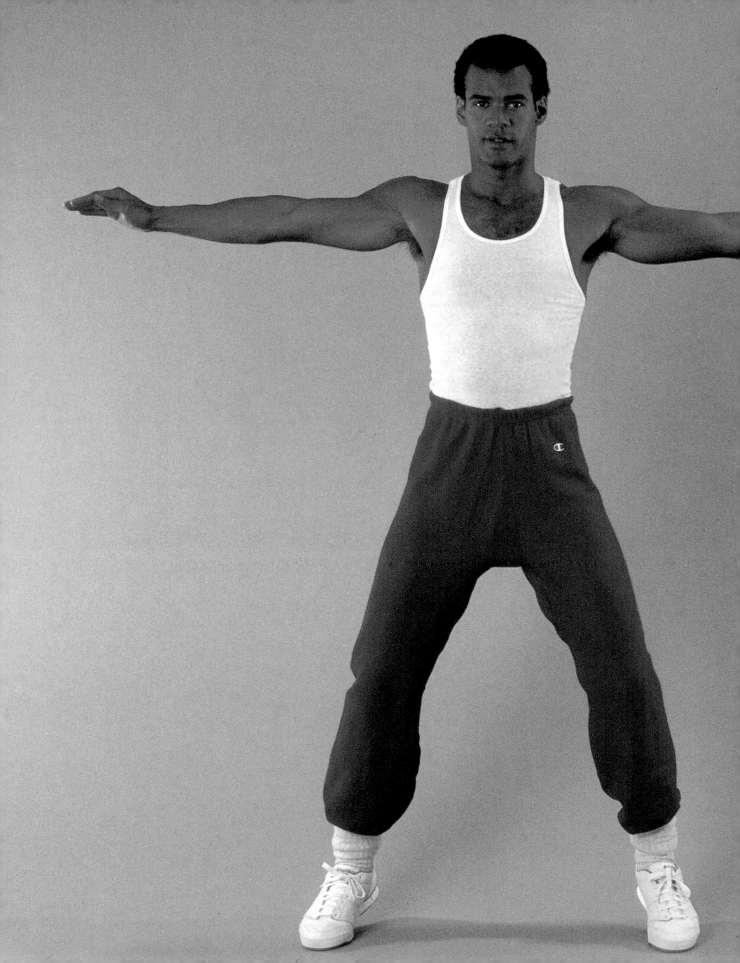

CHAPTER THREE

Aerobic Movement

*Out of the dance studios
and into the training programs
of professional athletes*

Aerobic movement combines choreographed rhythmic exercise with music. Dance steps incorporating jazz, ballet and disco are mixed with calisthenics, running and jumping for a workout that is varied and lively, whether you perform it in a class or at home. In recent years, aerobic movement has become the second most popular form of exercise in the United States, after walking. Although it was initially perceived as a women's sport, aerobic movement has made significant inroads with men. Professional athletes, including boxers and baseball players, were among the first to take it up, and it has since gained popularity with other men looking for an enjoyable way to get in shape.

Aerobic movement works the entire body with a variety of exercises that involve muscles in your arms, legs and torso. Many of the movements are drawn from other aerobic activities; yet aerobic movement does not restrict you to repeating a single motion. Your muscles and joints move through their full range of motion, building

Shoes designed for running or walking do not adequately protect you for aerobic movement. Running shoes are most heavily padded in the heel and have a wide outersole to prevent your foot from rolling sideways. But aerobic movement often involves landing on the ball of your foot and moving from side to side. Well-designed aerobics shoes, therefore, are cushioned in the forefoot and support lateral movement.

A new shoe should fit snugly and feel stable. If the uppers are of cloth or soft leather, they will stretch. When the uppers overlap the midsole by more than one quarter of an inch, it is time to replace the shoes. With heavy use, you may need to replace them every few months.

muscle endurance and enhancing flexibility in a way not usually found in single-movement activities like running and cycling.

Many people find that the music heightens their enjoyment and their motivation to exercise. Rock, folk, musical comedy, jazz and other types of music can all supply a tempo and a rhythm that will inspire you to move.

Not only is aerobic movement enjoyable, but it can also provide a cardiovascular workout on a par with bicycling and swimming. Although some low-level aerobic movement may not raise your cardiovascular function high enough for a training effect, it will improve your VO_2max significantly when done vigorously. One study found that a six-week aerobic movement program improved cardiovascular fitness as measured by an average 14 percent increase in the distance participants could run in 12 minutes and by a decrease in their resting heart rate of almost four beats. In another study, those completing a seven-week program showed increases in VO_2max comparable to participants in a jogging program. Other studies have reported such positive psychological effects as more self-control, higher alertness and improved ability to think clearly.

Many people join aerobic movement programs to lose weight. Assessments of its effect on body fat vary, however. Although some studies report that moderate weight loss occurs during an aerobics program, most studies show no change in body weight or body fat. Researchers have concluded that you cannot lose weight from an aerobic movement program unless you alter your diet.

Aerobic movement will tone your muscles. Since it provides a full body workout, it is particularly helpful in reshaping your body while you are on a reducing diet. In addition, it can give you a greater sense of coordination than most other aerobic activities.

A common misconception about aerobic movement is that it is injury-free. In fact, its free-form nature, variety of movements and the intensity of jumping expose the frequent participant to stress injuries. Your muscles and joints are not accustomed to many of the movements in an aerobics routine. And with the amount of hopping, twisting and jumping necessary for a productive workout, you will occasionally land badly. This has resulted in reported injury rates of about 40 percent among participants and up to 75 percent among instructors of aerobics. The majority of these injuries are minor and require no treatment aside from rest. Most complaints are similar to those of runners — shin splints, "runner's knee," metatarsal and arch pain, calf muscle stress and lower back pain. Many of these can be prevented by stretching, warming up and cooling down, and wearing shoes designed for aerobic movement. Barefoot exercisers sustain the most injuries, followed by people who wear running shoes.

A suitable surface is also important to cushion the impact as your feet land. Bare concrete or concrete covered only by a carpet is the worst surface for your workouts. The best surface is a hardwood floor suspended over a cushion of air. Though generally difficult to find,

Aerobic Movement Program Tips

◆ Ease into your routine: Your joints and muscles need to grow accustomed to the movements gradually. Alternate each exercise with a minute or two of walking or jogging lightly in place for the first few weeks. Shorten the periods of walking or jogging between exercises as your fitness improves, and gradually leave them out all together unless you need to catch your breath.

◆ Vary your routine to keep it interesting. If you like doing aerobics in groups, attend a class at least occasionally and adapt exercises you learned in class to your routine.

◆ Improve your posture by paying particular attention to your body alignment as you perform your routine. Imagine your spine as a stack of disks that you need to support by standing erect when you are upright and by controlling your movement with your muscles when you are bent. Do not train your muscles to support bad posture by hunching your shoulders or standing crookedly as you exercise.

◆ Make yourself a tape of music to fit the length of your routine. Choose music with a steady beat that inspires you to move. The music should have a suitable eight-beat rhythm — like most popular and country music — without irregular beats or sudden shifts in tempo. Fit the tempo to the exercise: The warm-up music should be slower than the aerobic phase, and the music to go with the cool-down and stretch should have a leisurely beat. To choreograph your routine like a professional, choose a new piece of music for each exercise.

this type of surface is used in most good dance studios. You can make any floor suitable by exercising on a dense rubber pad.

The threat of injury has led many people to low-impact aerobics; it entails more upper body exercises and dance movements that keep one foot on the ground at all times. At least one study has found that low-impact aerobics, with less jumping and skipping, makes it more difficult to raise your heart rate than does traditional aerobics; however, your oxygen consumption may be elevated enough to produce a training effect. For endurance training, it is important to check your heart rate frequently if you choose low-impact aerobics.

Part of the fun of aerobic movement can come from performing it with a group. When you enroll in an exercise class, choose a level that is comfortable for you and check the instructor's qualifications. (There are several national organizations that certify instructors.) Poor instruction — in a class or on a videotape — is one reason the injury rate of aerobics is particularly high. Excessively prolonged repetitions, high jumping or repeated patterns on one foot are among the movements that increase your risk of injury.

Clearly you will derive the greatest benefit and enjoyment from an aerobics program if you perform your movements safely. The following pages present a routine designed to build endurance safely while you have fun working out.

The Right Routine

A good aerobic movement routine works your body's large muscles, raises your heart rate and keeps it in the target zone for the duration of the workout — all without exhausting you. The half-hour routine here and on the following 10 pages is designed to do this. It begins with a five-minute warm-up followed by a 20-minute aerobic segment of arm, torso and leg movements. A five-minute cool-down ends the routine, and there is a special section on jumping rope, which can be substituted for the aerobic movement phase.

To avoid strain or overexertion, do each movement for the time specified rather than a set number of repetitions. Add repetitions as you get fit. For example, you might start out doing 30 body pumps in a minute and over a few weeks work up to 60. If you become tired in the middle of a routine, substitute walking in place for jogging or hopping.

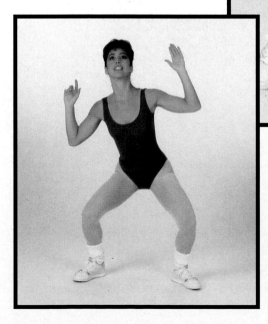

Warm-Up
. . . .

1 **THE BODY PUMP** From a standing position, lean on one leg and reach up with the opposite hand, stretching the muscles along your side *(above)*. Raise the heel of your free foot to protect your back. Shift over to the other leg by lowering your arm and squatting slightly *(left)*, which warms up your thigh muscles. Alternate pumping left and right for one minute.

2 **TWIST AND PUMP** With your arms at shoulder level, punch with one arm, gently twisting your torso and raising your heel *(below)*. Move into a squat *(right)*, then punch to the other side. Repeat the sequence for one minute.

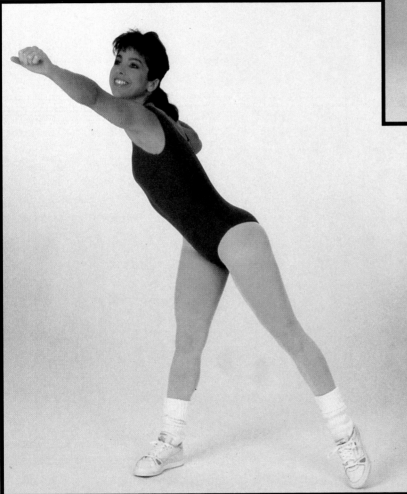

3 **MARCH AND HOP** March in place for one minute, raising your knees to hip level and swinging your arms back and forth to shoulder level *(below)*. When your fitness improves, add a low hop.

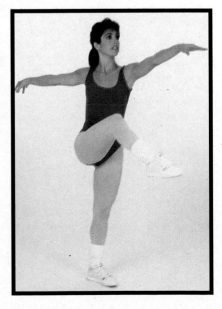

4 **THE JOG** To finish the warm-up, run in place for two minutes so you bring your heart rate into the target zone. As you run, swing your arms from the elbows. Protect your joints by landing lightly on the balls of you feet, then flattening your feet to distribute the impact.

Arms

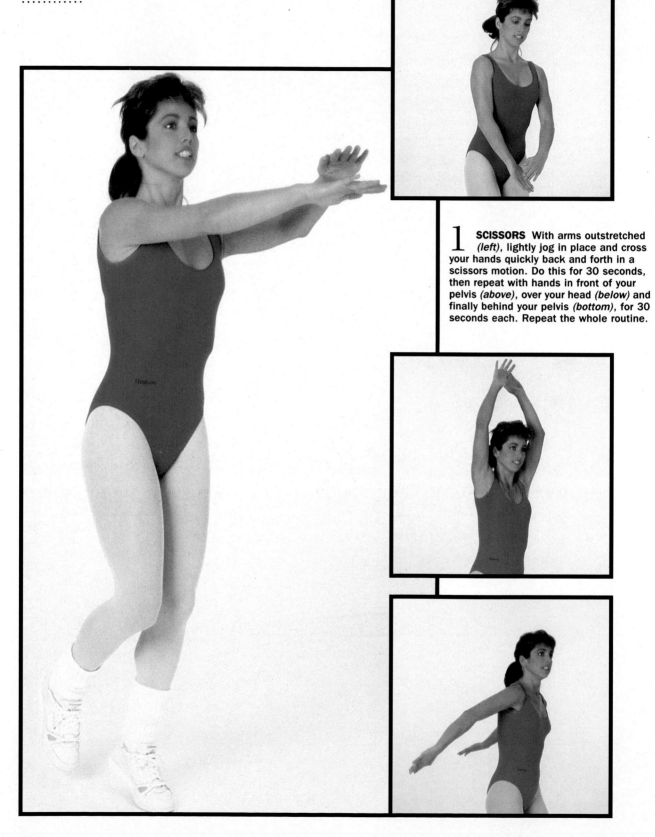

1 **SCISSORS** With arms outstretched *(left)*, lightly jog in place and cross your hands quickly back and forth in a scissors motion. Do this for 30 seconds, then repeat with hands in front of your pelvis *(above)*, over your head *(below)* and finally behind your pelvis *(bottom)*, for 30 seconds each. Repeat the whole routine.

2 **CHEST PRESSES** Raise your upper arms to shoulder level with elbows bent *(right)* and jog in place. Bring your arms together in front of your body *(below)*, then spread them again; briskly repeat this for 30 seconds as you continue to jog. Be sure not to let your arms sag. Repeat the routine. For the next set, start with your arms together, then raise them slightly *(bottom)*. Lower them to the starting position in front of your body. Repeat for one minute as you jog in place.

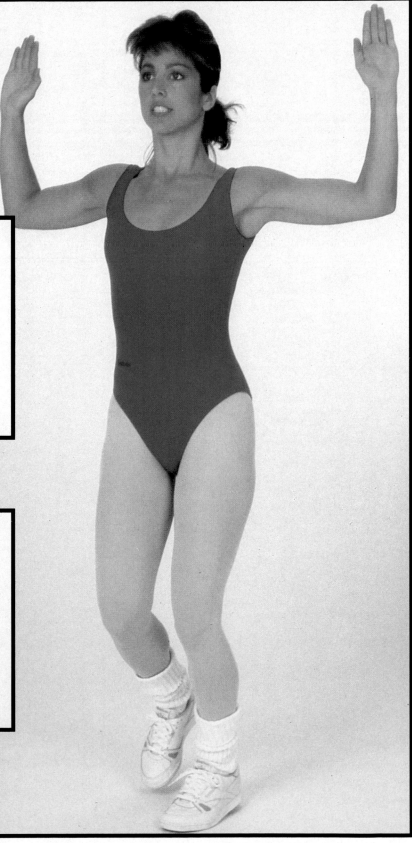

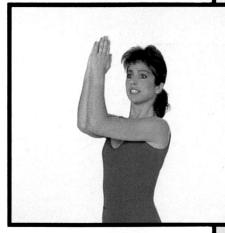

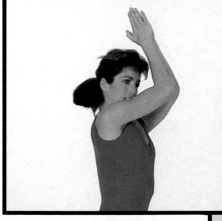

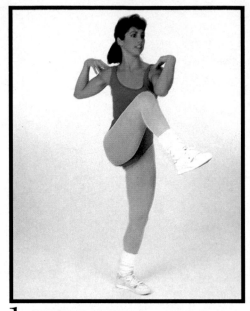

Torso

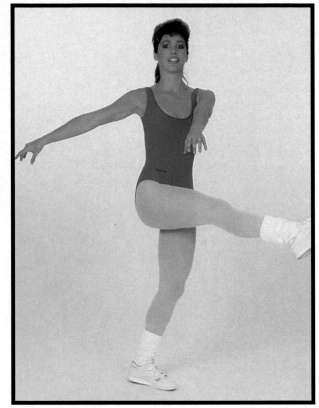

1 **HIGH KNEE LIFTS** Put your hands on your shoulders with elbows out *(above)*; lift knees in a marching rhythm for one minute, touching left knee to right elbow and vice versa. This exercise also helps firm abdominals.

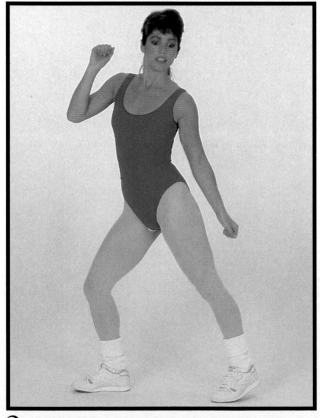

2 **LEG KICKS** Kick one leg across your body and hop on the other leg, can-can style, as you swing your arms in the opposite direction *(above)*. Alternate sides and repeat for one minute. For reduced impact, the hopping foot should flatten as it lands. Repeat for two minutes alternating kicks with knee lifts.

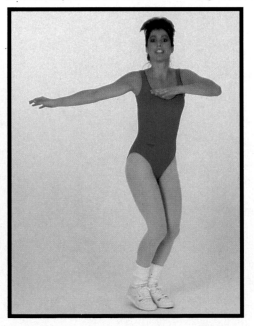

3 **TWISTER** With your feet apart, turn your body from side to side by raising your heels and twisting on your toes *(above)*. Swing one arm up, the other down. A more advanced version is the ski twister *(right)*: Hop with both feet, and swing arms at shoulder height from side to side. Perform for one minute.

Legs

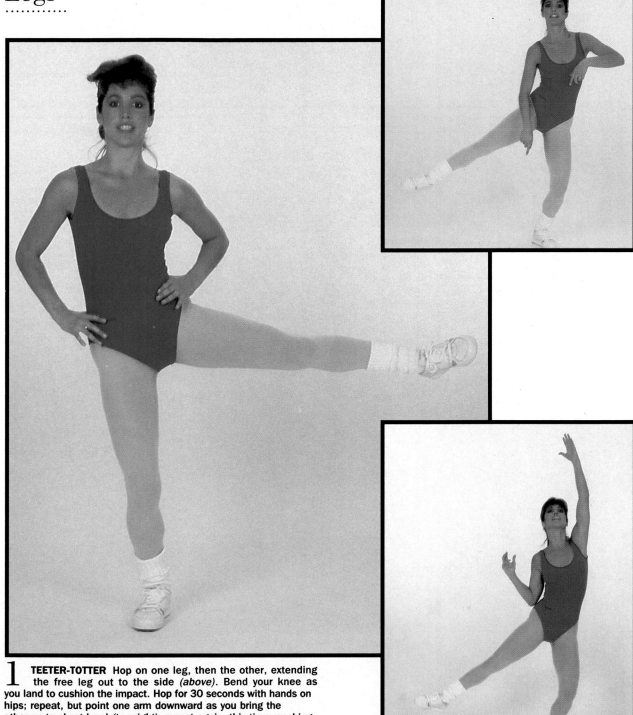

1 **TEETER-TOTTER** Hop on one leg, then the other, extending the free leg out to the side *(above)*. Bend your knee as you land to cushion the impact. Hop for 30 seconds with hands on hips; repeat, but point one arm downward as you bring the other up to chest level *(top right)*; repeat again, this time reaching up with each arm *(right)* for one and a half minutes.

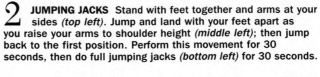

2 **JUMPING JACKS** Stand with feet together and arms at your sides *(top left)*. Jump and land with your feet apart as you raise your arms to shoulder height *(middle left)*; then jump back to the first position. Perform this movement for 30 seconds, then do full jumping jacks *(bottom left)* for 30 seconds.

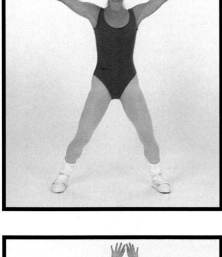

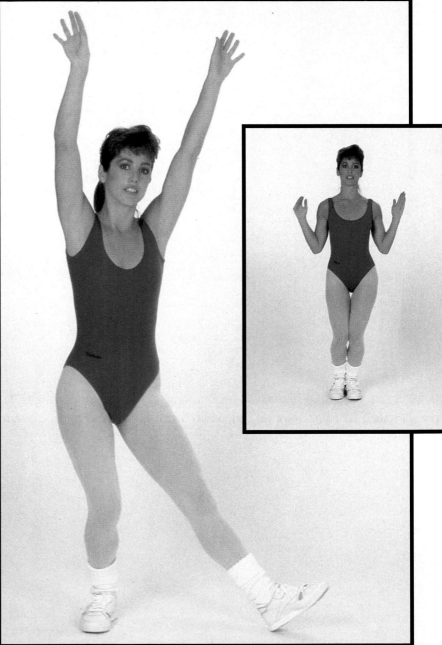

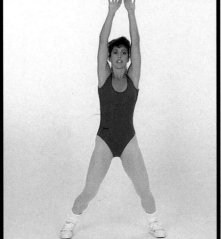

3 **HEEL JACKS—ARMS UP** Hop on one leg, and extend the free leg to the side with the heel on the floor; at the same time, raise your arms *(above)*. Hop again and bring both legs together as you pull your arms down at your sides *(inset)*; then hop with the other leg. Repeat for 30 seconds.

4 **HEEL JACKS—ARMS OUT** For 30
seconds, hop on one leg and throw
your arms out to the side at shoulder
height *(below)*. Then hop with both legs
together and fold your arms in from the
elbow *(inset)*. Repeat on the other side;
then alternate this exercise with heel jacks
— arms up *(opposite page)* for one minute.

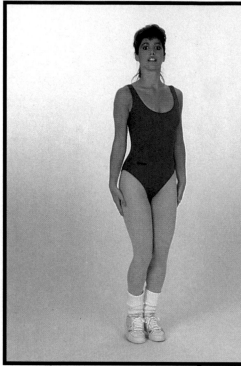

5 **LUNGES** Jump and turn to one side, raising your arms overhead *(right)*. One leg extends forward, the other behind; keep the heel off the floor. Then hop so that you face forward *(above)*, and jump to the other side. Repeat for one minute.

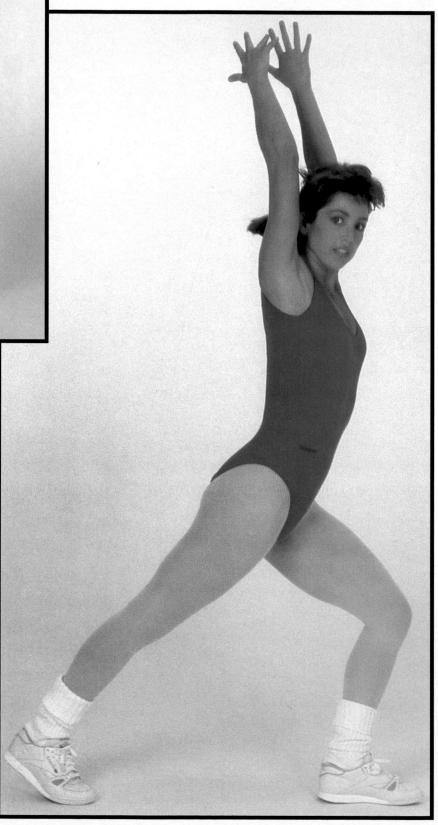

6 **LEG AND ARM** With arms bent at elbows, lift one knee to waist level *(right)*. Lower knee and raise both arms straight overhead *(below)*, then pull down arms to the first position as you lift the other knee. Repeat for one minute.

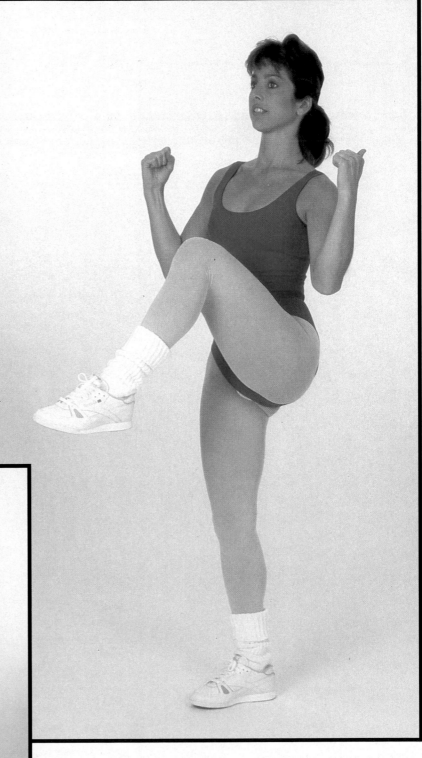

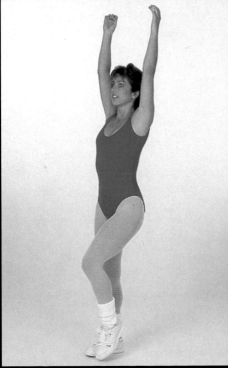

Cool-Down

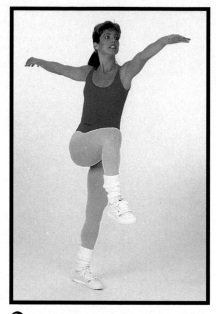

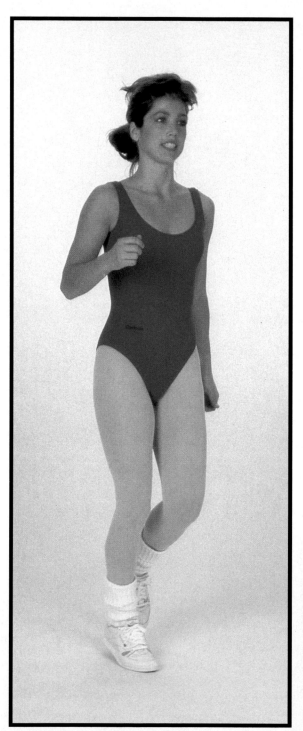

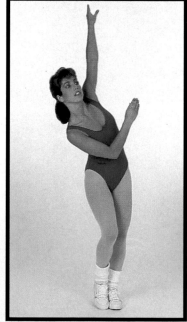

2 **THE MARCH** March in place for two minutes. Lift one knee hip high, then the other; at the same time, swing your arms back and forth to shoulder level. As you march, gradually slow your pace.

3 **BODY SWING** Standing with arms at sides, lean forward slightly and step from side to side for one minute. Swing arms in the direction you are stepping.

1 **THE JOG** Jog lightly in place or around the room for two minutes, swinging your forearms up and down. Flatten your feet on landing to cushion the impact. If jogging is too strenuous, walk.

4 **STRETCH** Finish the cool-down stretching to prevent stiffness and injury *(page 29)*; in particular, stretch the muscles of the lower leg and foot, where most injuries in aerobics occur.

Jumping Rope

For variety in an aerobic movement routine, you can jump rope. All you need are shoes suited for aerobics and a rope. The handles should reach your armpits when you stand on the middle of the rope. Jumping rope is also a good indoor substitute for the other exercises in this book.

Jumping rope should never be your only exercise, however, both because it is hard to sustain without becoming exhausted and because the range of movement is small: You use the same muscles continuously, but you do not fully extend or contract them.

Since jumping rope raises your heart rate fairly high, alternate 30 seconds of jumping rope with 30 seconds of light jogging in place for the first few weeks. Gradually build up to one-minute intervals, with 30 seconds of jogging in between, then two minutes of jumping and so on. To get the desired benefits and prevent injuries, you need not jump longer than 20 minutes. Be sure that you also warm up and cool down.

Begin a jump rope routine with a jogging jump *(above)*; hop from foot to foot for each swing of the rope as if you were jogging in place. At first add a rebound hop for each rope swing. As you improve your fitness level, swing the rope faster, jumping only once per swing. A more vigorous style is the two-footed jump *(left)*, which you can also do slowly or quickly. Because you land harder, however, you should jump no higher than one inch off the ground. Always land on the balls of your feet, with your knees slightly bent. Let your feet flatten to absorb impact.

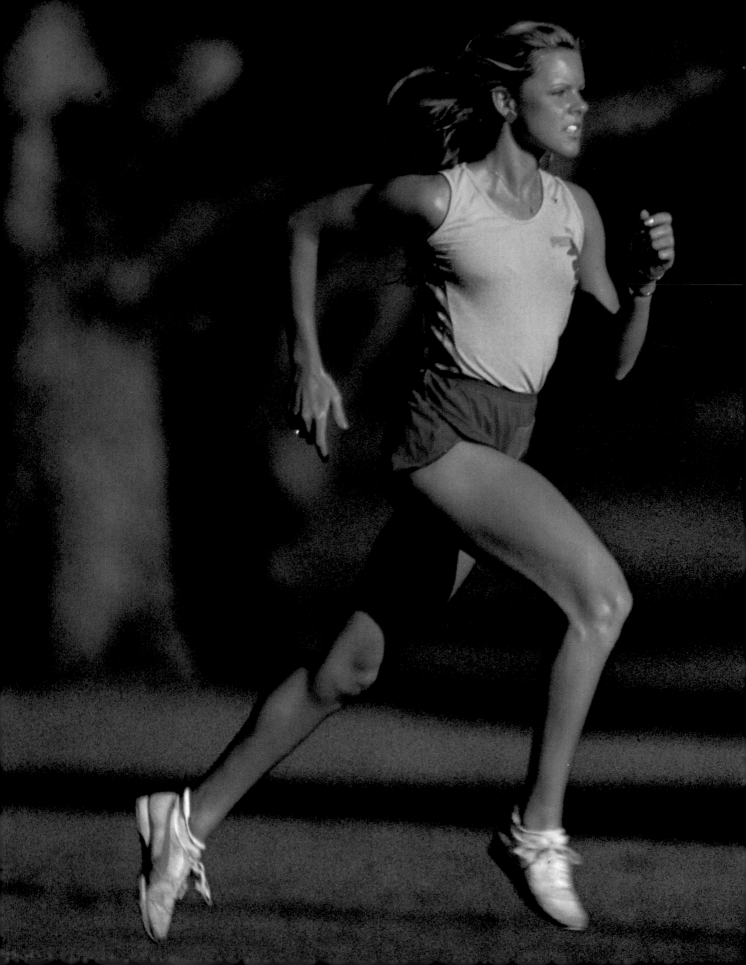

CHAPTER FOUR

Running

*The first exercise of the
fitness era: still the workout of choice
for 12 million Americans*

Distance running is a peculiarly human activity. Although other animals can easily outsprint us, we have an unusual talent for endurance. Navajo Indians can catch the pronghorn antelope, one of the fastest animals on earth, simply by running it down over great distances. Similarly, Australian aborigines can wear down kangaroo, and Tarahumara Indians chase deer through the mountains of northern Mexico until the animals collapse from sheer exhaustion.

Zoologists have observed that perhaps only horses, camels and certain dogs surpass us in endurance. But even horses may not be able to stay in front of a determined human. One of the longest horse races in the world, the 100-mile Tevis Cup in California, is usually won in about 14 hours, a time easily outpaced by top ultramarathoners.

What makes human physiology uniquely suited for long-distance running? Heat dissipation is the most important factor. Humans possess a cooling system that no other creature in the animal kingdom has. We sweat a lot, and because we are naked — or at least not covered with fur — our sweat can cool us very rapidly. We can keep going while most other animals, which rely on panting to cool themselves off, must slow down or stop to avoid hyperthermia, a rise in body temperature that can be fatal.

Our endurance talent is also made possible by our unusual breathing system. Most other running animals are quadrupedal — they have four legs — and their breathing rate is tied to their gait when they are trotting or galloping. The muscles and bones in their chest area must absorb the shock when their front legs hit the ground; therefore, they can take only one breath per gait cycle, which is not an efficient way to breathe for long-distance running. But because humans are erect and bipedal, our chest cavity does not have to contract and expand with each stride; we can breathe at whatever rate is most efficient for a particular pace.

Even our omnivorous diet, along with our metabolism, predisposes us to endurance running. Unlike animals, we have the power to alter our diets to fit our needs. Research has shown that a diet high in carbohydrates not only contributes to well-being and protects us against disease, but it may also enhance our ability to run long distances and pursue other endurance activities. This explains why athletes have shifted away from high-protein regimens to diets that emphasize pasta, bread and other high-carbohydrate foods. Humans also have unusually large thyroid and adrenal glands. During exercise, these glands may secrete increased amounts of the hormones that enhance our ability to use more glucose and fatty acids, fuels essential to meet the energy demands of long-distance running.

Although we live with the comforts of modern times, our bodies are still tuned for endurance running. This genetic predisposition to endurance activity may explain why so many sedentary and out-of-shape individuals adapt quickly to endurance running. Studies show that running can produce significant improvements in cardiovascular work capacity for almost everyone, including children and elderly persons. Even heart attack victims have taken up running programs, and some have completed 26.2-mile marathons and longer races. At the other end of the fitness scale, a survey of endurance athletes indicated that the average VO_2max of elite distance runners is higher than that of every other group, including world-class cross-country skiers, competitive rowers, competitive cyclists, elite swimmers and professional racquetball players. The same survey showed that runners have a lower percentage of overall body fat than any other group of athletes.

Many runners report that, along with its superb conditioning benefits, running also gives them a feeling of euphoria and well-being, the so-called runner's high. Although many nonrunners remain dubious about runner's high, a few studies indicate that running may actually stimulate the production of certain hormones called endorphins, which can alleviate pain and elevate mood. Some researchers have suggested that, for most casual runners, the mental uplift after a run is due not to

Fluid Replacement: Drink Before You Are Thirsty

When you run or perform any exercise intensely, you need to replace fluids lost through sweating. This is especially important in hot weather, when you can lose up to three quarts of water in an hour. Such extreme fluid loss can be accompanied by increased body temperature, lethargy, nervousness, thickening of the blood, and a decline in the ability to sustain exercise due to circulatory and cardiovascular deficiencies. In endurance events like marathon running, severe water deprivation has even caused death by heatstroke.

If you drink only when you are thirsty, though, you can get into trouble. Thirst is an indicator of the body's need for fluids, but studies have shown that runners and other athletes may ignore the thirst signal due to the strain or excitement of physical activity. It is possible, in fact, to lose up to two quarts of water before you are aware of fluid loss. Furthermore, thirst is quenched long before you have replaced the lost fluids. Experts have observed that if you relied entirely on thirst to rehydrate yourself, it might take you several days to reestablish the proper fluid balance. To maintain the proper balance, particularly in hot weather, follow these recommendations:

1. Drink before you exercise. Studies confirm that this keeps body temperature from rising and allows you to exercise more comfortably in the heat. One or two eight-ounce cups of liquid taken 10 to 20 minutes before your workout should be sufficient.
2. Drink while you exercise, preferably a cup or two every 20 to 30 minutes. Contrary to popular belief, this will not make you sick or hamper performance.
3. Drink plain water. It is absorbed more efficiently than anything else. Sports drinks are an acceptable alternative as long as their sugar content is low. Sugar hinders absorption, so avoid drinks that contain more than six percent sugar, which includes most soft drinks and many fruit juices. Avoid caffeinated drinks, such as coffee and tea, which act as a diuretic and may increase fluid loss.
4. Drink cool liquids. Research shows that they enter the digestive tract faster than warm ones. And there is no evidence that cool liquids cause stomach cramps or side stitches.
5. Drink at a water fountain along your running route; on a hot day you may want to carry a water bottle with you.
6. Drink after exercise. Again, water is the preferred fluid.
7. Weigh yourself. After prolonged exercise, this is the best way to be sure you are fully rehydrated.

endorphins, but to a greater sense of control over one s life that comes from engaging in an exercise program. Any euphoria that you experience, therefore, should simply be enjoyed as one of the many benefits that running offers.

Another significant advantage people see in running is its convenience. You can run almost any time, day or night, winter or summer. And you can run virtually anywhere: on a track, on city streets, down country lanes, through the woods. You can even run in place, although many people find that their interest and enthusiasm for running is in direct proportion to the beauty and variety of the passing landscape.

On the other hand, a common complaint about running is that it is monotonous, and in fact boredom is the reason most often cited for giving up running. But boredom is preventable. Studies show that people who give up their programs usually perceive them as tedious rituals that must be performed within a rigid framework. To help avoid this feeling, vary your running as much as possible. Run at different times of the day, along different routes and for different lengths of time. Let your mind wander. Runners who tend to dissociate, or daydream, while they run show greater adherence to their running programs than those who are excessively aware of minor discomfort and fatigue.

As long as you have a good pair of running shoes, you can run safely on almost any surface. Grass is the preferred surface of many runners because it is firm and supportive, yet softer and more yielding than most other surfaces. Few running experiences, for instance, match the exhilaration of slapping barefoot over a well-manicured golf

Common Running Surfaces

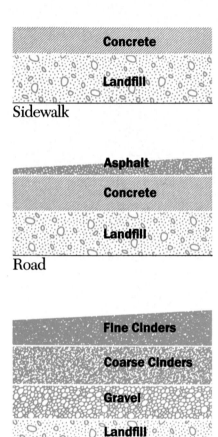

Sidewalk

Road

Track

Some running surfaces are better than others. Concrete — the material for most sidewalks — is made of stone and cement, and it provides little shock absorption for a runner. Roads paved with asphalt offer a softer surface that is preferred by many runners. More resilient still are cinder tracks, which consist of loose layers of crushed stone. You can run safely even on concrete, however, by wearing a good pair of running shoes.

course. Dirt roads and paths are also relatively soft and level, so these surfaces are popular among runners.

Most runners, though, spend the bulk of their running time on paved roads, simply because these surfaces are the most accessible. If you have a choice, run on asphalt instead of concrete. Asphalt has more yield and bounce than concrete, which makes it less stressful on the feet and knees. No matter what road surface you choose, be sure to alternate the side of the road you run on. If you stay on only one side, the banking of the road is likely to put added stress on the curbside leg, increasing the chance you will injure it.

A track provides a good running surface, but the repeated loops can be monotonous. Indoor tracks may be even more tedious — some of them require you to run 24 laps or more to the mile. Running on an indoor track can also lead to injury, since the continuous turns may strain the feet, ankles and knees.

Though running along a beach is tempting, you should not do it excessively. Soft sand offers little support, which may cause you to tire quickly or to develop cramps in your calf muscles. Running on the firmer sand near the water is much more comfortable, but the slope of the surface may overstress the seaside leg.

Except during dangerous storm conditions, the weather should never be an excuse for not running. Indeed, some of the great joys of running are to crunch over freshly fallen snow or to splash through a summer shower. Even on the coldest winter day, you can stay warm. Since the heat production of exercising muscles can be 15 to 20 times that of muscles at rest, your major problem in the cold may turn out to be overheating. If you overdress, your clothing will become damp with sweat. When you stop exercising or if a chilling wind draws heat from your clothing, you will suddenly become cold. And once both dampness and cold envelop you, it is difficult to recapture body heat: Wet clothing conducts heat from the body much faster than dry clothing. Therefore, in cold weather, it is best to dress as if it were 10 to 20 degrees warmer. If you feel a little chilly when you start out, you should be completely comfortable during the run.

To add to your comfort while running in the cold, wear a wool cap that you can pull over your ears. (You lose more heat through your head than anywhere else.) Also, wear light gloves, such as cotton gardener's gloves, or put socks on your hands. To avoid chafing and wind burn, rub petroleum jelly on your nose, chin and cheeks.

You can also run with comfort in the rain. To keep warm and dry, wear an undergarment made from any of the synthetic materials that "wick" away moisture from your skin. For outerwear, many runners favor athletic suits made of special fabrics that are water-resistant yet still breathable, allowing water vapor from sweat to escape but keeping out water droplets from the rain.

Many runners do not hesitate to run in the heat, but it is essential when doing so to observe common-sense precautions, particularly if you are starting a running program. Hyperthermia, or overheating, is

Running Program Tips

◆ If you have not run before, do not try to run hard or far the first time you go out. Begin by alternating five minutes of slow jogging and five minutes of brisk walking. Otherwise, your muscles, tendons and ligaments will become sore and stiff. Alternate walking and jogging for the first three or four weeks of your program, gradually increasing the jogging segments until you can comfortably run for the entire session.

◆ As you improve your cardiovascular fitness and condition your legs, do not be tempted to run too quickly: This is more likely to lead to injury than to fitness. Stay well within your target heart rate zone. If you are running at a good pace and still have enough breath to carry on a conversation, you are probably training at the proper intensity.

◆ Run for time, not mileage. If you aim to run three miles at each workout, you will probably run the same course again and again. Not only will you grow bored, but you may also try to run it as fast as possible, thus increasing your chance of injury. If you run for a set period of time, however, you can be creative about your route and maintain a reasonable pace.

◆ As you progress from one training level to another in your program, it is important that you do not increase your running time by more than 10 percent each week. If your total running time is two hours for Week A, for instance, add only 12 minutes at most to your running time for Week B.

most common among inexperienced runners. During the dog days of summer, avoid direct sun as much as possible; run in the early morning or after 6 p.m. But if temperatures are consistently in the 80s or 90s when you run, give yourself time to adapt. Keep running as frequently as you have been, but run for shorter periods and at a slower pace. Increase your time and pace gradually over two to four weeks.

To prevent overheating, expose as much of your skin to the air as possible. Merely sweating will not cool you off — the sweat must evaporate. Even a cotton T-shirt will slow the evaporative process. The ideal warm-weather running outfit consists of shorts, a sleeveless fishnet shirt and low-cut socks. Because you may sweat heavily, you need to drink before, during and after your run *(page 61)*.

The biggest aggravation runners face, however, is not the weather but getting injured. The most common injuries *(pages 70-71)* occur at the foot, ankle, shin, knee, hip and buttocks. Fortunately, most running injuries can be prevented. Wearing a good pair of running shoes is crucial, as is not pushing yourself too hard. Equally important is observing good running form, which increases the efficiency of running by reducing jarring up-and-down motions. Developing a natural, fluid style not only helps avoid injury, but it allows you to fully realize running's potential as a superb aerobic conditioner.

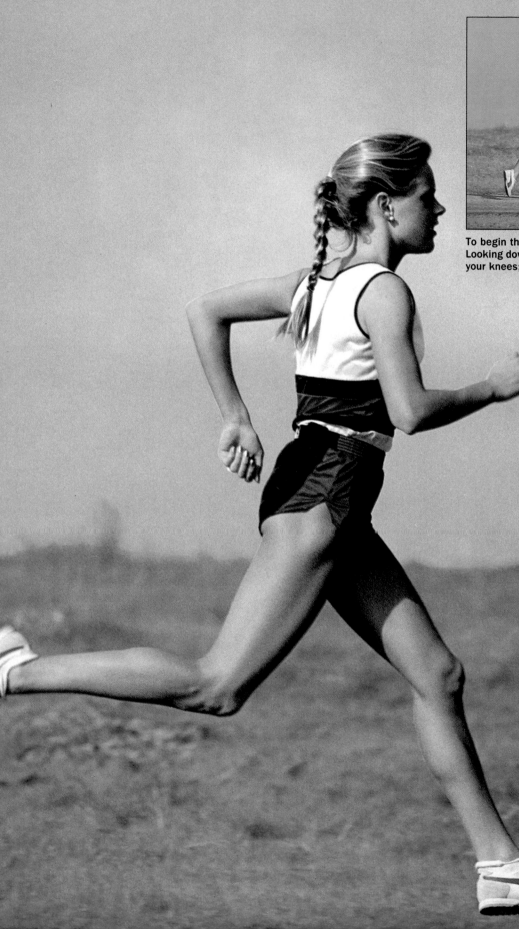

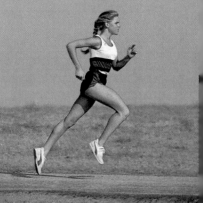

To begin the float phase, look ahead.
Looking down will shorten your stride. Lift
your knees; do not drag your feet.

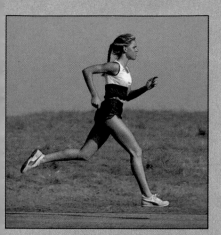

You should land with barely a sound. Quiet running indicates that you are moving efficiently, with little stressful pounding.

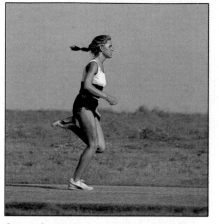

As your foot makes contact, your knee flexes like a coiling spring. Your footstrike should feel like a bounce, not a hard impact.

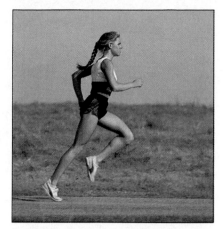

Roll forward on your foot, driving into the float phase from your toes. You should direct your bounce forward, not upward.

Proper Stride

Running for endurance is easier when you run with good form. To improve your form, concentrate first on stride.

Good stride consists of a fluid, continuous motion that, when taken apart as in the sequence above, is marked by two distinct phases: the float phase, when the runner is airborne, and the contact phase, when one foot is touching the ground. During the contact phase, the runner's leg both supports the body and drives it forward. Most runners spend about 40 percent of their time

To maintain a relaxed running style — the most important aspect of good stride — run with just a suggestion of forward lean (left).

airborne. The proportion of flight time reaches about 50 percent with increased speed.

To maintain a smooth stride, it is important first of all to stay relaxed. Running with fists tightly clenched and shoulders hunched will most likely cause tension and make your stride short and jerky. To keep your hands and shoulders relaxed, try touching your thumb to your forefinger or middle finger as if holding a dime. Concentrate on a smooth stride in which the legs reach a full, natural forward extension during the float phase. The knee should be flexed slightly as the foot strikes the ground.

65

Carriage and Footstrike

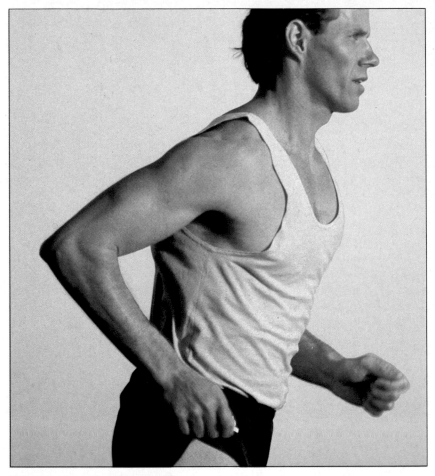

Keep your elbows bent at about 90 degrees. Dangling your arms or holding them to your chest will cause a loss of power in your stride. Your arms should move forward and backward, each arm and shoulder in concert with the opposite leg, your hands brushing your hips. Avoid excessive side-to-side arm movement, which tends to deflect energy laterally, away from the direction of travel.

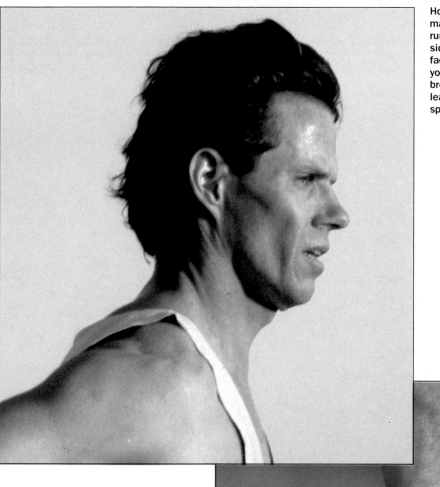

Hold your head high; it will help you maintain proper posture and efficient running form. Avoid bobbing your head from side to side, clenching your teeth or tensing facial muscles. Breathe normally through your mouth. Shallow, rapid or fluttery breathing restricts oxygen intake and can lead to side stitches — thought to be spasms of the diaphragm muscle.

A proper footstrike is more flat-footed than heel-to-toe. Land on the back of your foot but not on the back of your heel, which over time can cause injuries. As running speed increases, the point of first contact moves farther from the heel. You should land with the outer edge of the foot touching the ground first. Then the foot should roll forward diagonally, toward the big toe, smoothly distributing the impact.

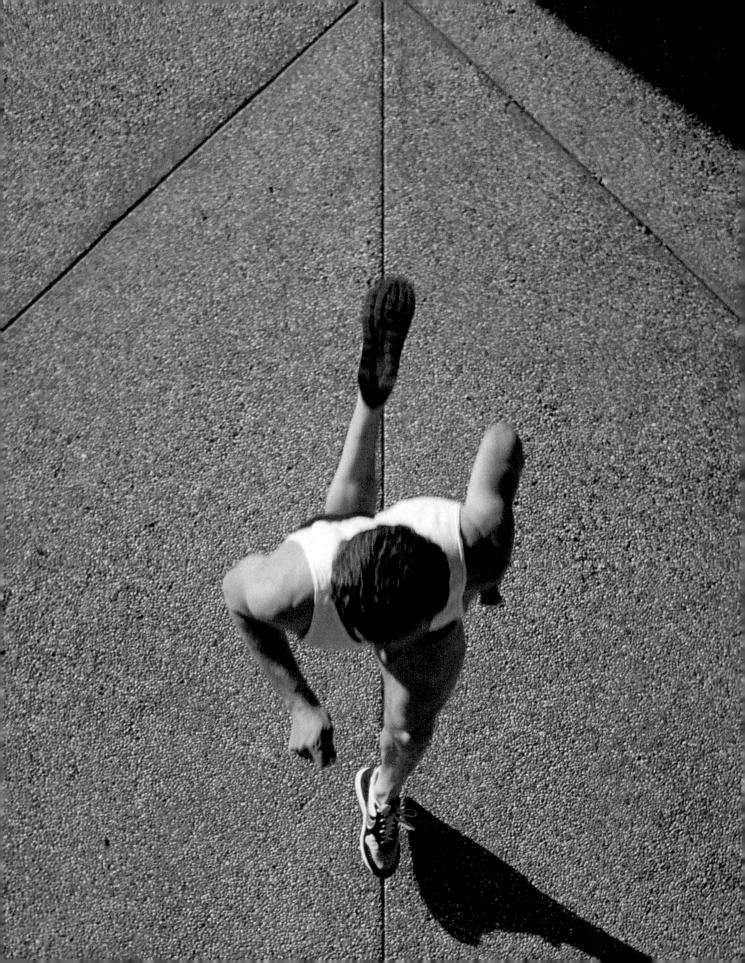

The Perfect Alignment

Symmetry is a major distinction between running and walking. When you walk, your feet land on either side of an imaginary line running in front of you, and your body's center of gravity oscillates back and forth over this imaginary line. No such swaying occurs in running. Your center of gravity should move as if in a channel directly over the line, as shown at far left. Likewise, your feet should land on top of the line every time they hit the ground. This alignment is important to running efficiently; no motion or energy is wasted in unnecessary lateral movements.

The simplest way of gauging symmetry is to be aware of your arm movements. If one arm swings out to the side more than the other, or if it crosses over the median line of your body, your form overall is probably unbalanced. A minor asymmetry may not matter: Even Olympic and professional runners often have slight irregularities in their form. But for less experienced runners, any noticeable deviation may slow them down, or even produce injuries by overstressing tendons and ligaments.

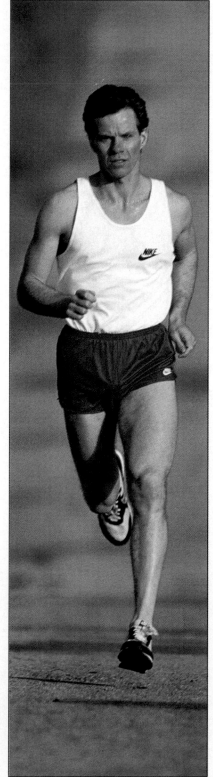

If your body is aligned properly, your feet will land on a line directly in front of you *(left)*. Even your nose will follow this line. A good way to check your alignment is to have a partner run behind you.

As your foot prepares to meet the ground, it turns in slightly *(right)*. In this way, your body is perfectly balanced in a straight line, from the nose to the foot, throughout the contact phase.

Preventing Injuries

When you run, your feet strike the ground anywhere from 800 to 2,000 times a mile, at a force of about three to five times your body weight. A runner weighing 160 pounds may cumulatively absorb about 280 tons of force per mile. It is no wonder, then, that running injuries are so common. According to one survey, about half a sample population of runners reported a running injury in the previous year that was serious enough to make them reduce training, take medication or see a health professional.

Most of the common runners' syndromes at right are overuse, or stress, injuries. Because they generally do not result in acute sudden pain, stress injuries can be insidious. Typically, you first feel pain from such an injury as you get out of bed in the morning, when the muscles are short and inflexible after a period of inactivity. The discomfort subsides as the muscles stretch with use during the day. The pain returns and becomes most severe at the beginning of a workout, diminishes during the run and then returns after you have finished running.

Much of the time, these injuries are the result of running incorrectly, and you can prevent them by observing good form. In addition, it is important that you build your program gradually and that you take the time to warm up and cool down properly. Also, wear a good pair of running shoes (*pages 72-73*).

If you do sustain an injury, it may very well respond to home treatment. To reduce pain and swelling, you can ice the affected area and take aspirin. Cut back or lay off your running during the recovery period. A chronic injury or any condition that results in severe pain should be diagnosed and treated by a physician.

Sciatic pain results from compression of the sciatic nerve by tight hip muscles or the lumbar disks. Discomfort is worst in the buttocks and thigh, but symptoms can also include numbness in the foot. Avoid strenuous downhill running.

Plantar fascitis and heel spurs are related injuries that involve painful inflammation of the plantar fascia — connective tissue along the sole — and its attachment to the heel bone. Run on soft surfaces and perform calf stretches.

Iliotibial band friction syndrome is an inflammation on the outside of the knee joint. It often begins as an ache but can progress to a painful burning sensation. Alternate the side of the road you run on.

Runner's knee, an aching or soreness around or under the knee, is caused by improper "tracking" of the kneecap. Avoid sprinting and excessive hill running.

Shin splints occur as pain or soreness in the shin region. They can sometimes lead to stress fractures. Run slower and on softer surfaces.

Displacement of the cuboid bone, a small bone of the ankle, is an acute injury that requires medical attention.

Stiffness or pain in the Achilles tendon is one of the most frequent runners' complaints. Avoid steep hills; do gentle Achilles tendon stretches frequently.

Choosing a Shoe

Look for a firm, durable heel counter; it will help stabilize the heel and prevent pronation, the tendency of the foot to roll in on impact.

Variable-width lacing holes accommodate wide or narrow feet. Lace only the inner eyelets if you have wide feet, the outer eyelets if your feet are narrow.

Some shoes have an external counter stabilizer that supports the counter and lends extra stability to the heel.

The lasting board, made of stiff cardboard or fiberboard, helps promote stability. It is just under the insole.

The arch cushion, a rubber insert in many good shoes, gives added arch support.

The midsole is the main shock-absorbing feature of the shoe; it provides most of the shoe's resiliency, but should not be so soft that the foot rolls or shifts on impact.

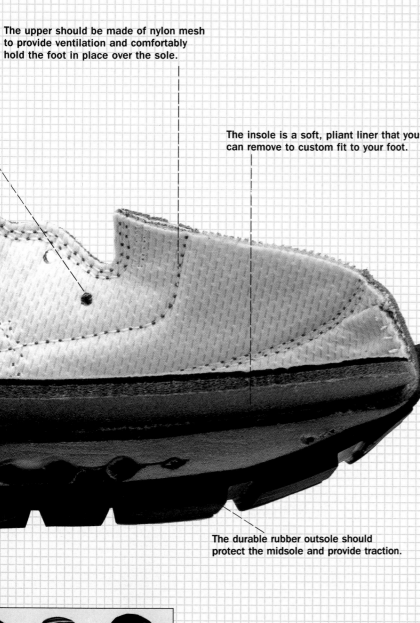

The upper should be made of nylon mesh to provide ventilation and comfortably hold the foot in place over the sole.

The insole is a soft, pliant liner that you can remove to custom fit to your foot.

The durable rubber outsole should protect the midsole and provide traction.

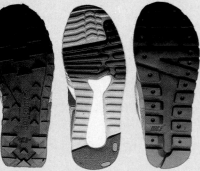

Look for center-depressed outsoles, higher on the outside than in the center, because they add stability. The waffled or ribbed bottoms are specially designed for traction, but any design is suitable for most running surfaces.

A running shoe is a specialized piece of equipment designed to stabilize the foot and to provide resiliency, or bounce, on impact. In choosing a shoe, many people assume that the more expensive it is, the better it withstands the repeated force of impact. Yet studies show that regardless of the design of the shoe, the materials used or its price, all running shoes lose about 25 percent of their resiliency after only 50 miles of running. Top-of-the-line models may be superior in certain respects, such as the stability they provide your feet, but they wear out at about the same rate as less expensive models. Replace your shoes when the heel counter starts to collapse or when the shoe feels "dead." Do not wait until the outersole is worn out. The midsole will have lost its resiliency long before then.

The most important qualities to examine in a new running shoe are flexibility and heel support. Check for flexibility by pressing on the heel and toe. The shoe should bend at the ball of the foot. If it bends too easily, the shoe may not provide enough cushioning. If it bends with difficulty, it will impede the natural flexing of the foot while running. Also, check to make sure the heel counter is solid and provides firm support.

When trying on running shoes, you should make sure that they fit snugly, firmly gripping your heel yet giving your toes plenty of space — at least half an inch — to wiggle. And good running shoes do not need to be broken in; you can run right out of the shop in them.

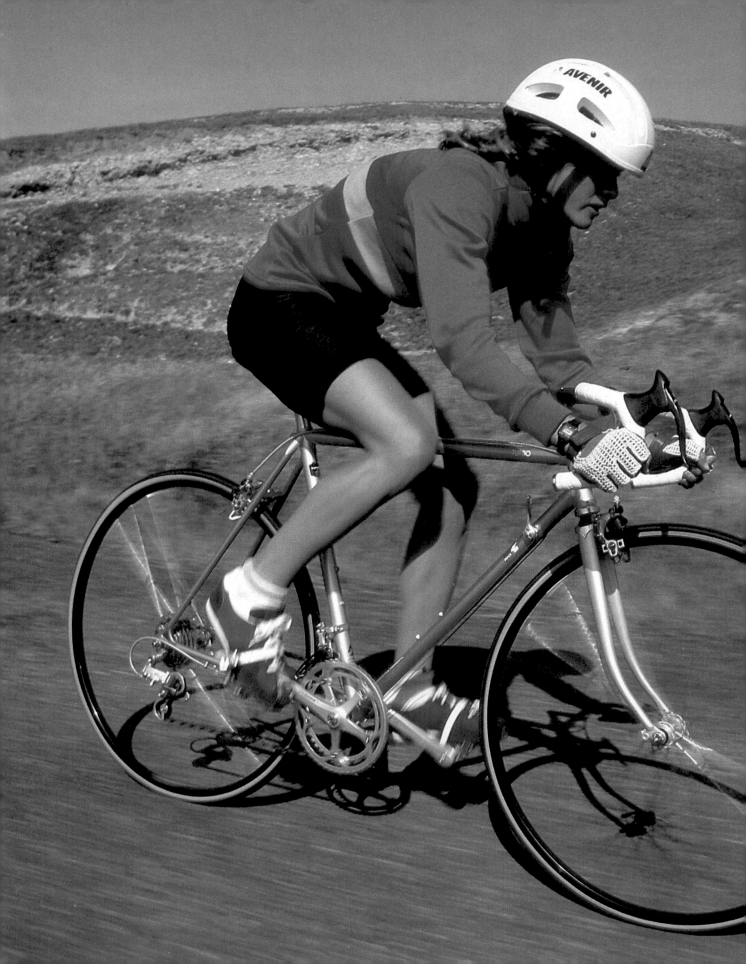

CHAPTER FIVE

Cycling

*Impact-free aerobic exercise combined
with the joy of the open road*

Like running, cycling is an exercise powered primarily by the great muscles of the legs. But while the runner launches himself into the air for a portion of each stride, becomes airborne and then strikes the ground, the cyclist uses his energy for forward propulsion only. In doing so, he avoids the stressful pounding of running that can lead to injury: The up-and-down, piston-like motions of the cyclist's legs are translated by the bicycle's pedals, gears and wheels into a continuous fluid drive.

On level terrain and for short distances, you can use any type of bicycle for exercise. But riding over hills or in stiff winds on a bicycle with only one or even three gears will be difficult. A 10- or 12-speed bicycle with downturned, or dropped, handlebars gives you a wider range of choices for regulating how hard and how fast you must pedal, and it allows you to maintain a regular cadence — the frequency at which you pedal — despite changes in wind direction and incline of the road. The demands on your cardiovascular system remain constant, which is essential to maximize fitness. With dropped handlebars, you can exert extra pressure on the pedals and gain more power in your cycling by using the various handgrip positions for leverage. You can also lean forward over the bicycle so that your arms absorb a significant amount of road shock. (In a more upright position, this stress is absorbed entirely by the spine.)

Cycling on a 10-speed can be running's equal as an aerobic conditioner. In one study that compared running and cycling during a 20-week endurance training program, cycling was at least as effective as running for developing cardiorespiratory fitness.

A Belgian study also confirmed that running and cycling programs are equally effective in developing aerobic capacity. However, when the investigators compared echocardiographs — cardiac images produced by ultrasonic waves — of cyclists and runners, they discovered that the cyclists had significantly greater heart-muscle mass. The reason, they theorized, is that cyclists not only power the bicycle with their legs, but they also use their upper bodies to help steady themselves in the saddle and transmit extra drive to their lower bodies. Gripping the dropped handlebars for leverage, cyclists in effect perform isometric exercises with their arm and shoulder muscles, strengthening and toning these muscles and further conditioning the heart. On the average, cyclists have better-proportioned upper body builds than distance runners. A study of Olympic athletes, for example, determined that the average cyclist's build was similar to the average swimmer's.

Along with these conditioning benefits, cycling also offers considerably more variety and mobility than either walking or running. Since cyclists routinely travel two to three times as fast as runners, they can observe more changing scenery and have the opportunity to visit more distant locations.

Cycling does, however, have a few drawbacks. While it is inexpensive in the long run, the start-up costs are high: At the very least, you need to buy a good 10- or 12-speed bicycle with toe clips and a hard-shell bicycling helmet (*pages 84-85*). You also need to consider location. Cycling for fitness in stop-and-go city traffic is difficult, while cycling over hilly terrain in the country may be too strenuous at first. Ideally, you should start out on relatively flat stretches of paved roadway. Weather can also pose problems. Rain can hamper your cycling by limiting both your vision and the effectiveness of your brakes. Ice and snow make cycling even more hazardous.

Another potential hazard is traffic. Although bicycling is generally a safe activity, more than 1,000 people die every year in the United States as a result of cycling accidents. In a survey of bicycling accidents in one middle-size city, researchers found that many of the automobile-related injuries were caused by drivers who failed to see the cyclist. In addition to wearing a helmet, therefore, you should wear bright clothing, obey traffic regulations, ride defensively and avoid cycling at night.

Cycling Program Tips

◆ For the first few weeks of your cycling program, cycle on terrain that ranges from level to gently rolling. Keep to a cadence of about 55 to 60 revolutions per minute (rpm), which should allow you to ride in low to moderate gears without straining.

◆ As your fitness improves, increase your cadence to about 70-80 rpm. This faster rate of pedaling may cause you to bounce in the saddle at first. If this does occur, cut back slightly on your rpm by shifting to a higher gear and work on perfecting your riding technique so that you can pedal smoothly at a rapid cadence.

◆ As you become stronger and better conditioned, try climbing long hills once or twice a week. Downshift as you approach the hill, not when you are on it. Climb at an easy pace until you develop a feel for how much effort it takes to reach the top. Learn to alternate sitting and standing out of the saddle while maintaining a constant pedaling effort.

◆ When bicycle touring, the duration of your workout is longer, which indicates that your intensity level should be lower. Therefore, you need not work continuously at your target heart rate: Strive for a heart rate of about 60 to 70 percent of your maximum and a cadence around 70 rpm. Brief periods of coasting can help you stay fresh and relaxed; extended coasting, however, breaks the rhythm and may induce muscle stiffness. Stand on the pedals to relieve saddle soreness and to stretch out your back and shoulders. Turn your head from side to side to loosen your neck muscles. To allay fatigue, keep your body limber by using the grip positions shown on pages 82-83.

Stress injuries among bicyclists are relatively minor. They consist mainly of tendinitis in the ankle region, "runner's knee" from too much hill work, sore shoulders, numb fingers and saddle soreness. Many of these conditions can be prevented or minimized by cycling with the proper technique, wearing proper clothing and using the right equipment. Cycling shoes, for instance, stabilize the feet in the clips and help prevent excessive rotation of the foot. Special cycling shorts padded with a chamois in the seat can prevent or reduce saddle soreness. Cycling gloves offer padded palms for shock absorption.

You should wear clothing that is comfortable and that does not bind or restrict blood flow. Clothes should not be so loose, though, that they can get caught in the spokes or other moving parts of the bicycle. In colder weather, wear layers of clothing so that you can peel off a layer or two as you warm up. Some cyclists slip a few sheets of newspaper between their outer layers of clothing and then, as they warm up, get rid of the newspaper.

Bicycle touring adds considerable enjoyment to a cycling program. You should build up your endurance with regular workouts, however, before attempting day-long outings. Most reasonably fit cyclists can comfortably manage day trips ranging from 50 to 100 miles.

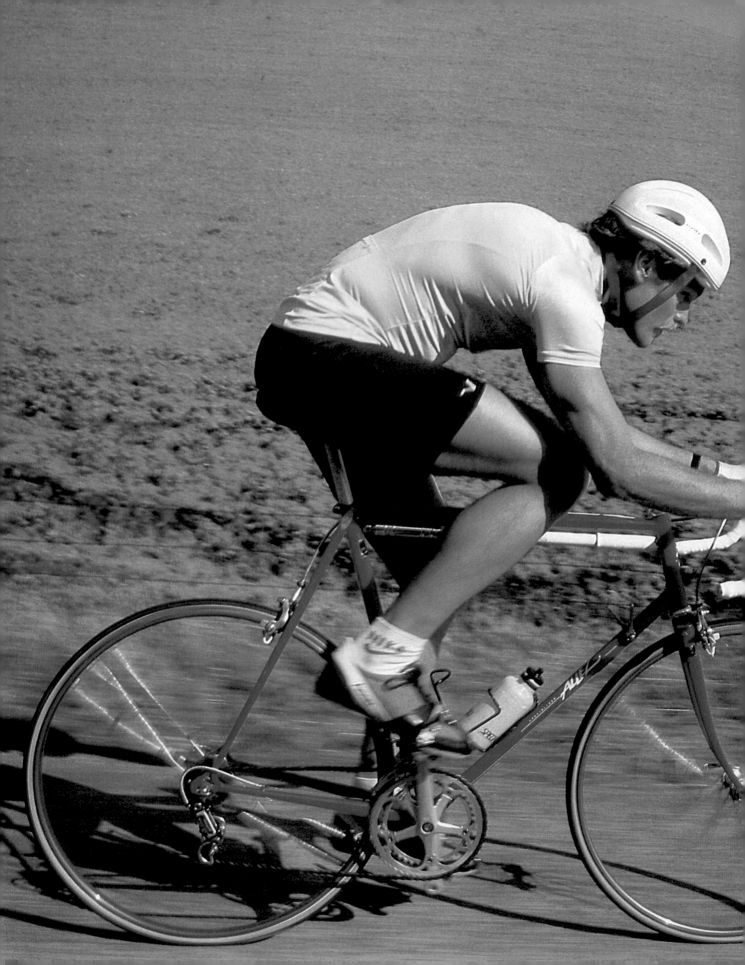

The Right Posture

To ensure good posture, you must choose a bicycle that fits you. If the frame size is too large or too small, the bicycle will be uncomfortable to ride and you may feel muscle soreness in the neck and lower back. Standard frame sizes range from 19 to 25 inches. To determine the right size, measure your inseam and subtract nine to 10 inches. When you straddle the bicycle, the top tube should be about an inch lower than your crotch.

Two other critical measures are the saddle and handlebar positions. Set the saddle height by having a friend hold the bicycle stationary while you sit on it. Place your heels in the pedals and backpedal. If the saddle height is correct, you will be able to backpedal with only a slight bend in the knees at the bottom of

Bend so that your torso and your upper legs form an angle of at least 45 degrees. Keep your knees inside your elbows.

the stroke. Too much of a bend means that the saddle stem is too low, and you will wobble and lose stroking power when you cycle. If the knee does not bend or if you have to reach for the pedal, then the saddle stem is too high and you will stress the knee joint. Keep the seat level or tilt it up slightly. Adjust the handlebars to 1-1/2 to 2-1/2 inches below the saddle. To check on the right handlebar height, ride with your elbows bent and your hands just below the brake levers. Look down at the front wheel hub. If you cannot see the hub because the handlebars are in the way, then your handlebar position is correct.

When you ride, bend from your waist. Do not slouch; your back should be relatively straight. This posture will afford you a relaxed and streamlined position without restricting your lung capacity. Also, be sure to keep your elbows bent to help absorb road shock.

Taking Hills

When you cycle uphill, lean farther over the handlebars to give yourself better forward momentum. Be sure to continue looking straight ahead, not down.

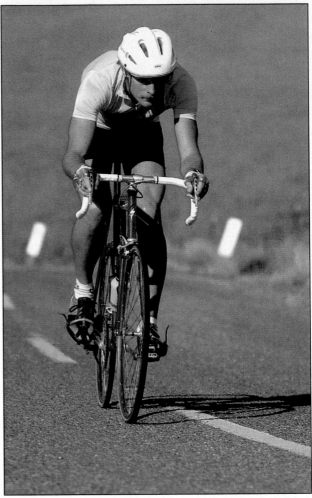

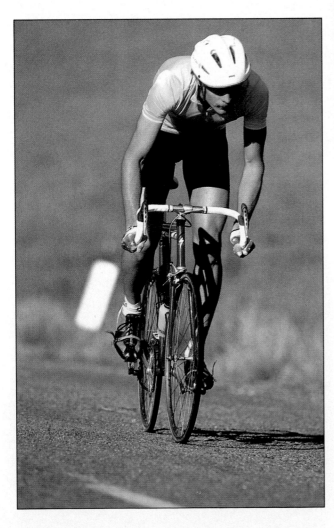

For steep hills that require extra effort even in the lowest gears, rise out of the saddle so that you can throw your whole body weight into each downstroke.

Cadence and Gearing

Inexperienced riders often believe that pedaling in high gears provides the greatest benefits because you have to push harder. They are wrong. Although your bicycle will go farther for each turn of the pedal, the intense effort can drain energy too quickly and even lead to injury. Experienced cyclists usually pedal at a high rate but in a low gear, a technique that gives them the most power and produces the least fatigue.

You should aim for a regular cadence between 70 and 80 rpm. To determine your rpm, you can count your pedal turns for 10 seconds and then multiply by six; for a more precise measurement, you can install a tachometer on your bike.

Choose the gear that best allows you to maintain your cadence and keep your heart rate within its target range. Shift gears so that your exertion level and cadence remain constant over varying terrain and during changes in wind direction. On an uphill stretch, for example, shift into a low gear to reduce muscle fatigue and stress on the knees. When going downhill, do not coast if you can help it, but shift into a high gear. This will not only help you maintain your rhythm, but also will make your bicycle more stable on the descent. Generally, if your legs get tired before you run out of breath, then you are in too high a gear; if you are breathless but your legs are still strong, then your gear is too low.

To add up to 30 percent more power to your stroking, think of your pedaling as not just an alternating push-down motion, but a continuous pull-up, push-down cycle. Your legs should work like pistons, keeping constant pressure on the pedals and toe clips, and driving the pedals both up and down.

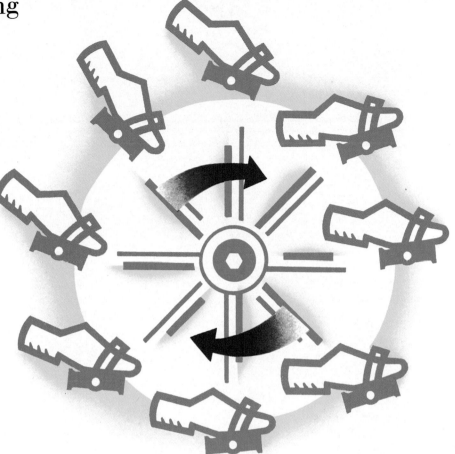

Your pedals should have toe clips and straps so that you can utilize the full 360-degree pedaling motion. To begin the downstroke, the ball of your foot applies pressure on the pedal at the 12 o'clock position and continues pushing to the 6 o'clock position. This is the strongest portion of your stroke, since part of your body weight combines with the effort of the quadriceps muscle to power the pedal down. The upstroke, which takes over at the 6 o'clock position and continues back up to the 12 o'clock, is not quite as powerful as the downstroke, but it conditions the opposing hamstrings and gives your cycling extra power.

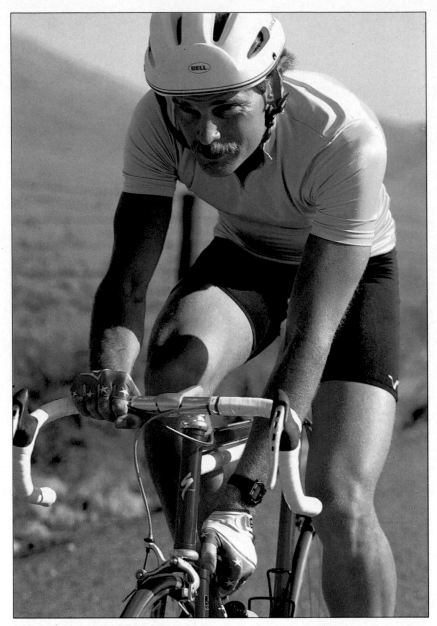

Gripping the Handlebars

The downturned handlebars on a 10-speed offer a variety of handgrip positions for shifting gears, adjusting your posture and giving your hands a rest.

In every grip position, bend your elbows: You will get better leverage and muscle power for pedaling. Your arms also become shock absorbers for your body when the bicycle hits bumps or potholes.

When slowing down on paved roads, use the front brake, which has the most stopping power. Apply steadily increasing pressure; clamping the brake suddenly may cause the wheel to lock. The rear brake should be used less for stopping than for keeping the bike from skidding. While braking, slide back in the seat to shift your center of gravity to the rear. This will prevent your being thrown over the handlebars.

On long rides, change your hand position often. Alternately relaxing some muscles and working others is the best way to avoid neck, lower back and wrist soreness.

When you change gears, get into the habit of moving the left gear lever with your left hand and the right lever with your right hand. If you use one hand to move both levers, you may bump the wrong lever as you reach over it to shift the other.

Position your hands near the handlebar stem before you shift gears
or signal turns. When you take one
hand off the handlebars, you will still have
control over the bicycle.

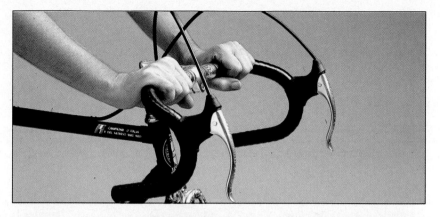

Grip the tops of the handlebars to bring your
torso more upright — a good restful
position for cycling along a flat road or
down a moderate incline.

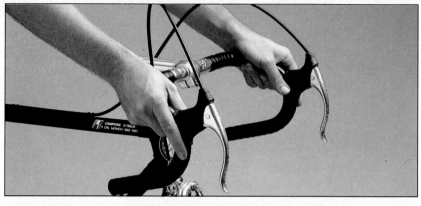

Rest your hands on the tops of the
brake hoods to increase support for your
upper body and to gain better leverage for
climbing hills.

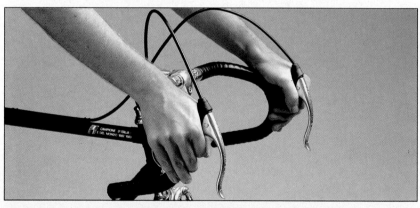

Put your hands in the drops — the grip
below the brake hoods — for braking and
when you are pedaling hard.

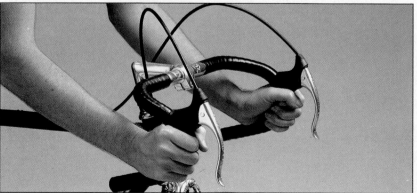

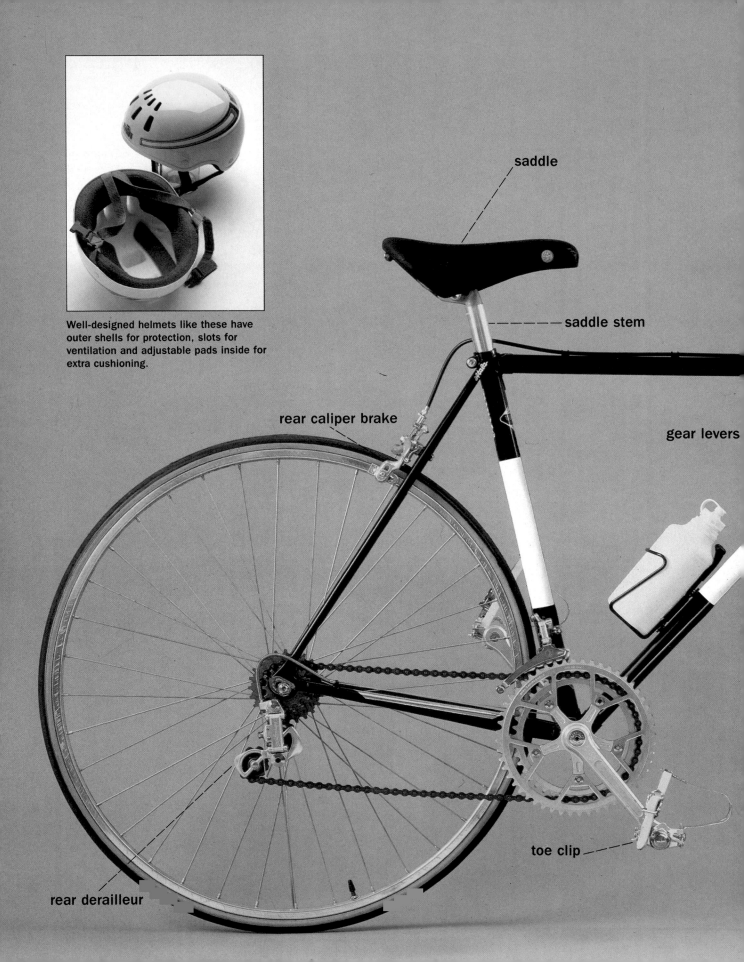

Well-designed helmets like these have outer shells for protection, slots for ventilation and adjustable pads inside for extra cushioning.

saddle

saddle stem

rear caliper brake

gear levers

rear derailleur

toe clip

Choosing a Bike

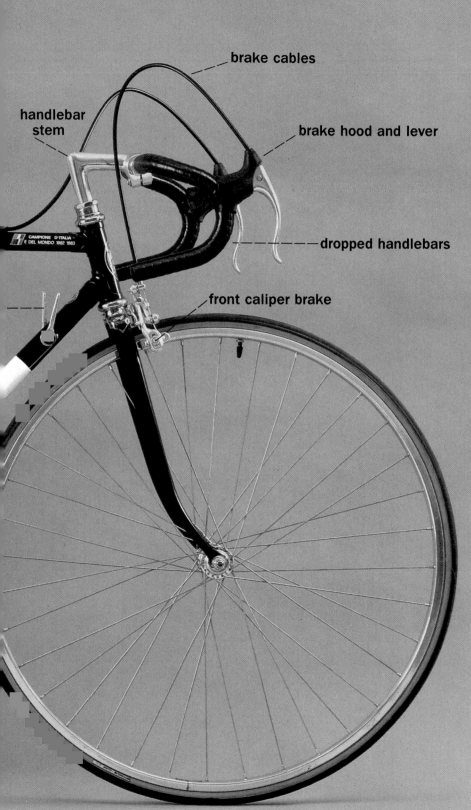

brake cables

handlebar stem

brake hood and lever

dropped handlebars

front caliper brake

For the best durability and responsiveness in a 10- or 12-speed bicycle, look for a bike made from either aluminum or chrome molybdenum, a light steel alloy. The frame tubing should be butted — thicker at the joints than in the center — for greater strength and lighter weight. Alloy wheel rims are also light yet strong. Look for a front wheel that has a quick-release mechanism for easy removal. Be sure the rear gearing mechanism, called the derailleur, is made of corrosion-resistant aluminum alloy.

Sidepull caliper brakes are generally stronger and more responsive than centerpull brakes. Good sidepulls have a release lever so that the brake will open and allow the wheel to be removed.

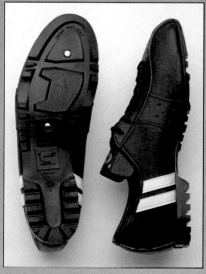

The soles of these cycling shoes have grooves that grip the pedal like cleats. Unlike cleated shoes, though, these are comfortable to walk in.

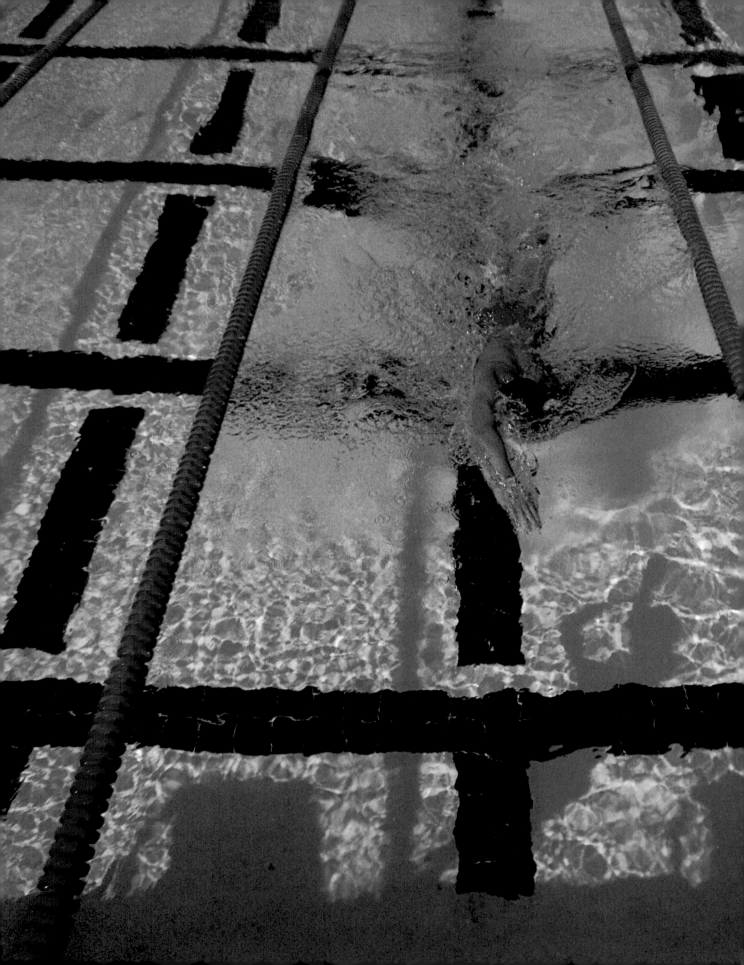

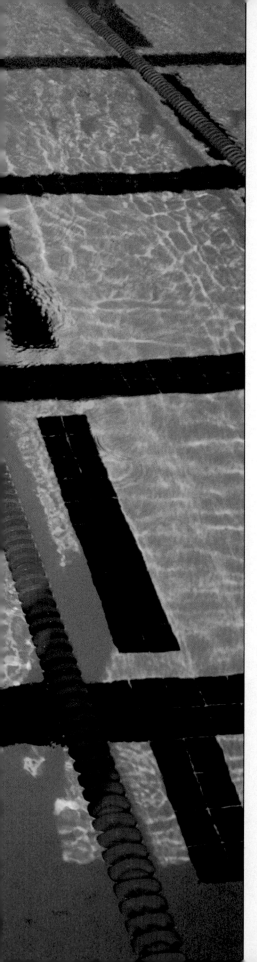

CHAPTER SIX

Swimming

*The best all-around exercise for the
least fit and the fittest*

The rhythmic movements of swimming place a demand not only on the heart and lungs, which help build endurance, but on virtually all the body's major muscle groups. As it develops muscle strength and endurance, swimming puts less stress on the body's tendons, ligaments and joints than running and other endurance activities.

Swimming's power as an aerobic conditioner at both beginning and advanced levels is well established. In one study, a group of adolescent women starting a swimming program raised their average VO_2max by 14 percent in just seven weeks. Among athletes, the average VO_2max value of top swimmers is almost on a par with that of runners and cross-country skiers, and slightly greater than that of cyclists.

Along with its training effect, swimming can condition the muscles of the upper body superbly — something running cannot do. Since the leg muscles are used mainly to keep the body level in the water, not for propulsion, the more a swimmer relies on his arms, the more efficiently he will move through the water. In fact, studies show that among competitive swimmers, about 80 percent of the forward motion comes from the arms and shoulders. Swimming is particularly effective for developing the chest and abdominal muscles. And because of controlled breathing, it further conditions the respiratory muscles and improves forced vital capacity, a measure of breathing ability.

The low injury rate among swimmers is due to the natural buoyancy of water, which holds the body up and relieves it of weight-bearing stresses. Since swimming does not place a burden on the spine, hips, knees and other joints, it is especially beneficial for people who are overweight and for those with knee or lower back problems. Because of the reduced stress, these people can work out longer and harder while swimming than while performing virtually any other type of exercise. Swimming is particularly effective for maintaining and improving the aerobic capacity of injured runners and other athletes who would not otherwise be able to work out.

To begin a swimming program, you must first find a suitable pool. In the United States, there are more than 2.5 million public and private swimming pools. Although competitive swimmers like to train in Olympic-size pools, many beginning swimmers find the 50-meter length of these pools daunting. In any case, most pools — even some advertised as Olympic-size — are a more manageable 25 meters (or 25 yards). You should try to avoid pools shorter than 20 meters; you will have to turn frequently, reducing the intensity of your workout.

The pool should have gutters to cut down on wave action and lane buoys or painted lines on the bottom to guide you. The ideal water temperature for a workout is around 80° F; in warmer water, you expend too much energy throwing off the heat generated by exercise.

You can get a satisfactory workout simply by swimming continuous laps in a pool; if you are happy doing this, by all means continue. But many people lose interest or fail to improve substantially if they repeat the same workout week after week. One way to vary a swimming program is with "broken swims," a training technique suitable for swimmers at all levels. This entails resting between each lap or set of laps, usually for a minute or less, so that you can recover oxygen without your heart rate falling far below its target zone. By changing the length and frequency of these rest periods, you can control your progress, as described in the box on the opposite page.

You can monitor your heart rate during the rest periods between laps. However, do not use the same target heart rate formula when you swim as when you perform land exercise. Studies have shown that heart rates remain naturally lower while swimming than while exercising on land. This is partly because your heart does not have to work as hard to keep your body temperature stable while you swim as it does when you exercise out of water. For swimming, subtract your age from 205, rather than from 220, and multiply the remainder by 65 percent and by 85 percent to determine your target heart rate zone.

Since water is constantly washing over you and cooling you as you

Swimming Program Tips

◆ Begin your program by swimming 100 meters — four laps in a 25-meter pool — with a one-minute rest period between each lap. As you gain confidence and swimming ability, gradually increase the number of laps you can do continuously. For example, a workout in the second or third week might consist of swimming 50 meters with a one-minute rest, then two 25-meter swims with a one-minute rest after each and finally another 50-meter swim. (This can be written in shorthand as 1×50, 2×25, 1×50.)

◆ To build endurance, shorten the rest period and increase the length of your continuous swim. For example, you might swim a sequence of 1×25, 1×50, 1×75 with 30-second rest periods, then repeat the sequence, for your workouts during one week. The following week, do 1×50, 1×75, 1×100, and shorten the rest periods to 25 seconds. As you build your aerobic base, try taking a particular distance — say 700 meters (28 lengths) — and breaking it into segments. These can be of equal size, such as 7×100, or you could swim seven laps, then six laps, on down to one lap, separating the segments with 15- to 30-second rest periods.

◆ A more rigorous variation is "pyramids," a series of laps in ascending and then descending number. You can swim a mile, for example, in a "pyramid eight": one lap followed by a rest period, then two laps, and so on up to eight, then back down (in shorthand, just remember 1-2-3-4-5-6-7-8-7-6-5-4-3-2-1). At the height of the pyramid, you should feel close to fatigue; as the numbers decrease, you will feel stronger and can even increase your swimming intensity.

◆ You can build both endurance and speed with interval training, which consists of a timed swim alternating with a timed rest. For instance, if you can swim 50 meters in less than one minute, give yourself intervals of 1 minute 15 seconds. Swim 50 meters as fast as you can, then rest for the remaining time: If you swim the 50 meters in 50 seconds, you have 25 seconds to rest. String your interval swims together for an interval set, for example, 4×50. The interval rest period encourages you to swim faster, giving you more time to rest; yet the rest period is short enough that your heart rate will not drop out of its target zone.

swim, you can sweat a great deal and not know it. Be sure to replenish this lost fluid by drinking a cup or two of water before you go in the water, every 20 to 30 minutes during your workout, and again when you have finished. You can also eat before you swim. It is a common belief that eating before swimming will cause severe stomach cramps; yet no research has ever proved this. In one study, swimmers ate a meal at intervals of one-half hour to three hours before a strenuous swim. None of the swimmers reported nausea or stomach cramps during or after the workout.

If you are a beginner, swimming lessons are worthwhile, and even intermediate swimmers can benefit from brushing up on their technique. An inefficient stroke makes swimming both awkward and harder. A smooth stroke makes swimming not only a perfect exercise, but also a perfect way to relax.

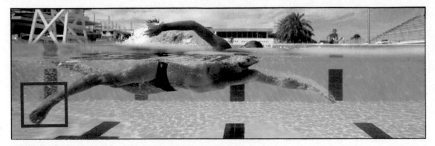

The flutter kick, highlighted at left, is used not so much for propulsion as for stability and balance. It keeps your body straight and your legs from sinking.

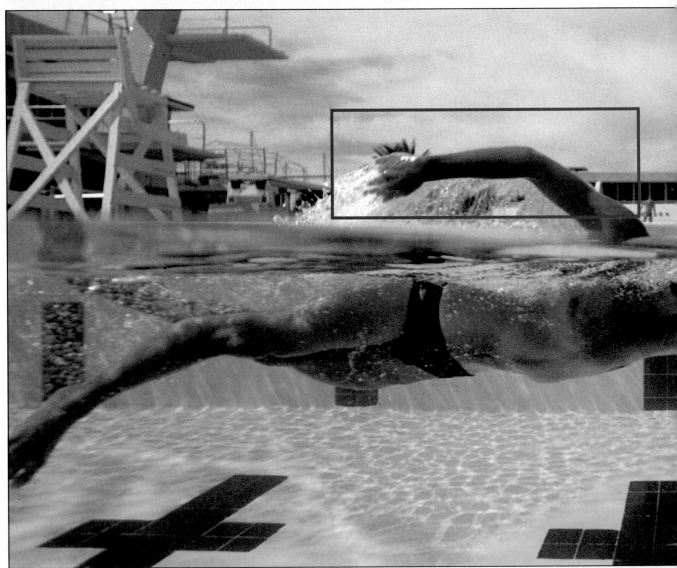

For efficient breathing in the crawl, you should roll your head to the side to inhale, rather than lift it out of the water.

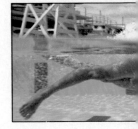

About 80 percent of the crawl's propulsive force comes from the arm stroke, highlighted below. Throughout the stroke, your elbow should be higher than your hand; this provides more power, and also reduces water resistance.

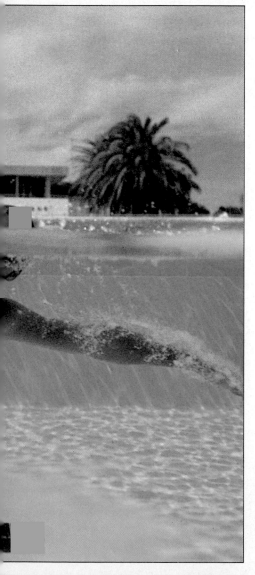

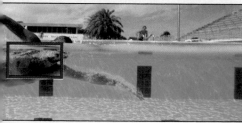

The Crawl

To swim for fitness, the most efficient stroke is the familiar front crawl, or "freestyle," as it is called in competitive swimming. Little energy is wasted in performing the crawl, and its constant, steady movements supply the proper rhythm for an aerobic workout. Less time is spent gliding with the crawl than with the sidestroke and the breaststroke. Unlike the butterfly stroke, the crawl does not demand bursts of energy that can quickly fatigue the swimmer.

The front crawl involves three basic elements: kicking, breathing and the arm stroke. The pictures here and on the following pages are not intended to teach a nonswimmer how to swim. Rather, they show how to swim for aerobic benefits, so that you can improve your technique. With fewer strokes per lap, you can cover more distance with less wasted energy.

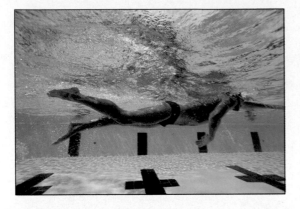

The Flutter Kick

A good flutter kick should "boil" the water, not splash it. To accomplish that, power your kick primarily with thigh and hip muscles, not calves and ankles. Bend your knees only slightly on the downkick and keep your ankles flexible. You should kick just deep enough — about 12 to 18 inches — to keep yourself stable in the water; kicking more vigorously will tire you out without moving you through the water much faster. Many swimmers are most comfortable with a rhythm of three kicks for each arm stroke.

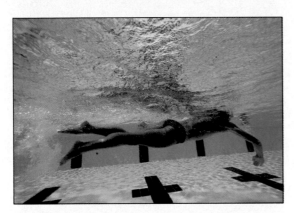

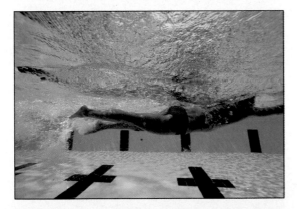

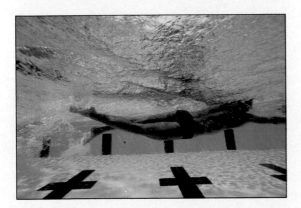

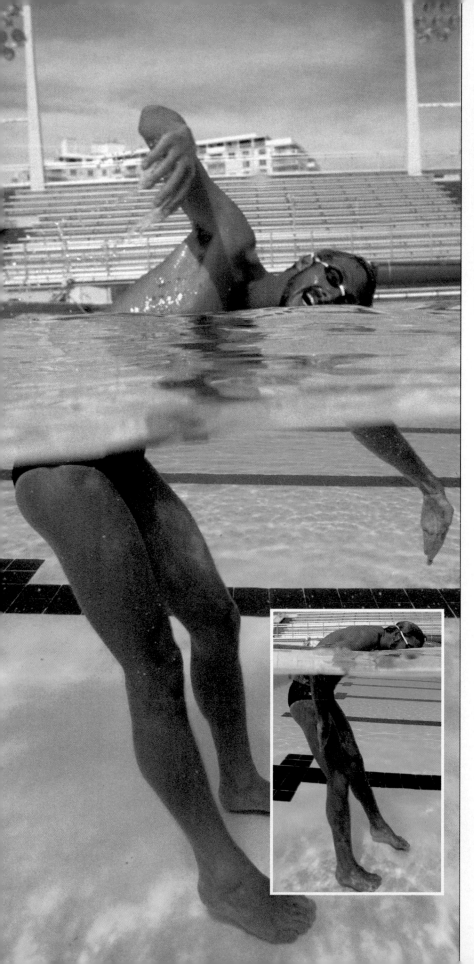

Breathing

Because it involves coordination of the head, shoulders, arms and respiration, breathing is often the most difficult aspect of the crawl to master. A good way to perfect breathing is to practice in waist-deep water. Place your face and shoulders in the water so that the water line is just above your eyebrows. Exhale slowly into the water. At the same time, pivot your head — in this example, to the right — and draw your arm out of the water as shown. As you go through a complete stroke cycle, your head should roll, turning just enough to take a breath of air. Be sure not to hold your breath; you should be exhaling or inhaling continuously. Practice this routine, pivoting your head either left or right, whichever feels the most natural.

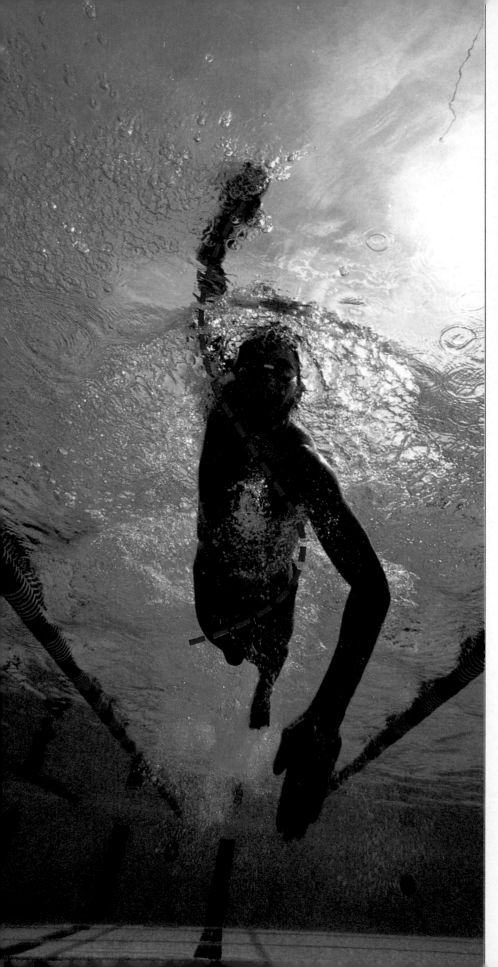

Arm Pull

To make the crawl stroke most efficient, your arm should sweep through the water in a figure S: It will then be pushing against still water, not water that is already moving backward and reducing the thrust of the stroke. Your hand should enter the water at arm's length directly in front of your shoulder. Bend your elbow so that it forms a 90-degree angle by the time your arm is halfway through its pull. During a stroke with your right arm, your hand should track in an S curve that goes underneath the right side of your face, across the left side of your chest and out past the right side of your lower torso. If you perform this correctly, you will never be flat in the water. Your body will roll from side to side so that you are swimming from shoulder to shoulder, which not only improves stroking, but provides more lift.

Arm Recovery

After completing the arm pull, lift your arm out of the water with the elbow slightly bent (1). Lead with your elbow and keep your hand close to the water. At the highest point in the recovery (2), your elbow should be bent at about 90 degrees. Reach forward (3) with your thumb turned downward. Your hand should enter the water at a 45-degree angle (4) with the fingers slightly spread, not cupped.

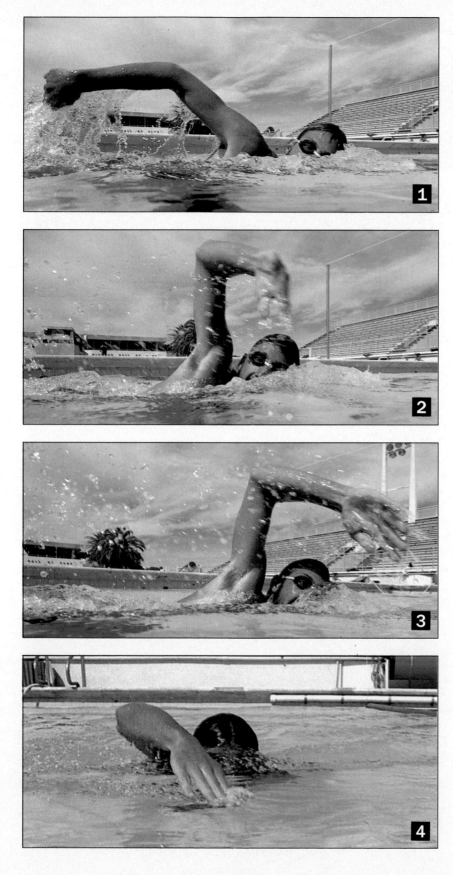

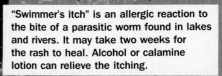

"Swimmer's itch" is an allergic reaction to the bite of a parasitic worm found in lakes and rivers. It may take two weeks for the rash to heal. Alcohol or calamine lotion can relieve the itching.

Swimming Ailments

Among swimmers, layoffs due to injuries are rare, which is one reason that swimming is such a good choice among all the aerobic activities.

Still, water sometimes harbors potential infections and causes irritations that can lead to layoffs just as surely as injury. Pure water is harmless, but a swimmer can sweat up to three pints of perspiration into a pool per hour. Perspiration provides a breeding ground for microorganisms. Chlorine and other chemicals cut down on the growth of microorganisms, but these chemicals can cause eye problems and dry out the skin and hair.

Swimming in open water also poses hazards. These include sunburn from prolonged exposure to bright sunlight, eye irritations due to debris in the water, and infections and stings from various organisms.

Some common swimmers' ailments are shown below, along with tips on how to avoid them or treat them.

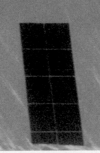

Many swimmers get sunburned on their shoulders and backs. To prevent sunburn, apply a water-resistant sunscreen with a sun protection factor of eight to 15.

Hair can dry out and become brittle due to chlorine or the drying effects of salt. Wash and condition your hair after each swim.

Chlorine can cause corneal swelling. Your eyes can also be irritated or damaged by sand or microorganisms in open water. To avoid problems, wear goggles.

Wet ear canals make ideal cultures for bacterial and fungal infections. Dry your ears after each swim. Ear drops containing alcohol help dry the ear canals.

"Swimmer's shoulder" is an inflammation of the soft tissues around the shoulder joint, causing diffuse pain. This condition can strike swimmers who use hand paddles. The cure: a few days' rest.

The pull-buoy and kickboard below help you refine your swimming technique. You can swim with your arms alone using the pull-buoy — two plastic cylinders joined by an adjustable tether. Place the buoys between your thighs, one cylinder on top, the other below. To build up your legs, use the kickboard: Hold it in front of you to support your upper body as you kick.

The hand paddles at left provide more resistance — and therefore can offer greater conditioning benefits — than the perforated pair above. But the perforated paddles are less likely to strain your shoulder muscles.

Swimming Aids

Many swimmers will find that the equipment on these pages can enhance their workout, their technique and their enjoyment of the water. Goggles protect your eyes from chlorine in a pool and help you see better in the water. They can even be worn over contact lenses. However, goggles often fog up when you swim. To prevent this, you can wet the inside of the goggles with saliva or apply a commercial defogging preparation.

Bathing caps keep hair out of your eyes, help to minimize water resistance, insulate your head in cool water and protect your hair from the drying effects of chlorinated water.

Kickboards, hand paddles and pull-buoys are training gear that you can use to isolate muscle groups for specific conditioning. Do not train with such devices for an entire session; instead, work with them periodically to give your workout diversity and a change of pace. Kickboards help strengthen your legs while pull-buoys have just the opposite effect — they support your legs so that you can work on your arm strokes.

You can also improve stroking technique with hand paddles. By increasing resistance to your arm movements, the paddles strengthen your shoulders, chest and arms. And they help you track your stroke through the water to achieve maximum power.

Goggles come in a variety of styles and tints; the pair at top has anti-fogging lenses. When shopping for goggles, place a pair over your eyes without attaching the strap. Press firmly and release. If they stay in place for a few seconds, the goggles fit.

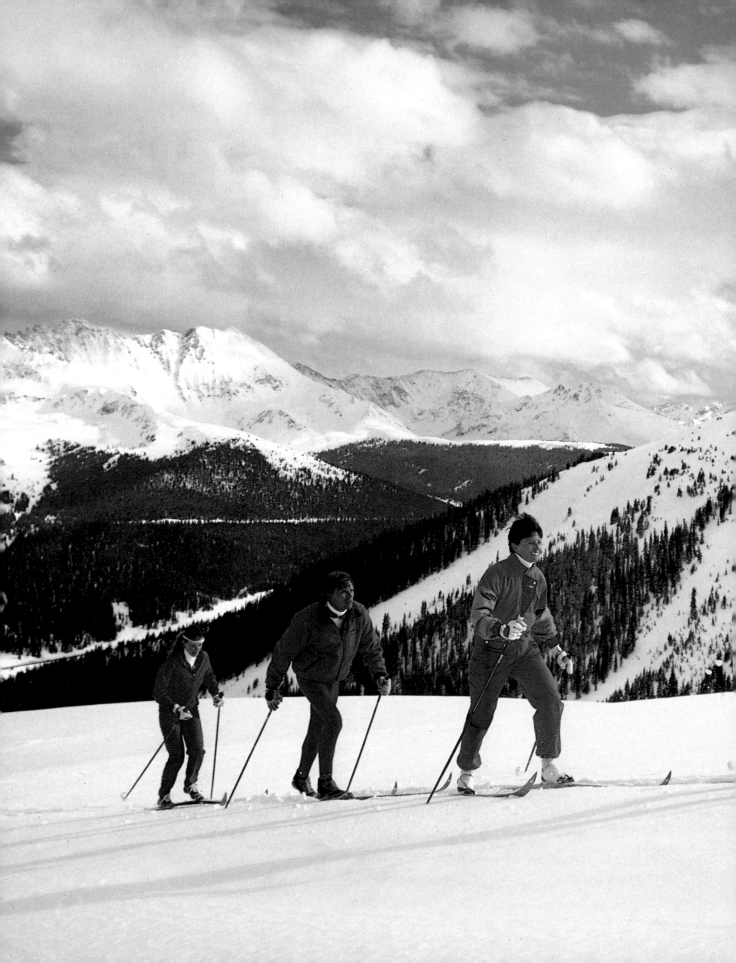

CHAPTER SEVEN

Cross-Country Skiing

The top-of-the-line workout that uses more muscles than any other endurance exercise

Performed at a training level and with the proper technique, cross-country, or Nordic, skiing is among the most demanding of endurance activities. Unlike downhill skiing, in which participants rely mainly on gravity, cross-country skiing requires the skier to propel himself about 80 to 90 percent of the time. And in contrast to running, swimming and cycling, cross-country skiing uses muscles in the arms, legs and trunk in nearly equal measure. Because of their collective need for oxygen during exercise, these muscles can make the heart and lungs of a cross-country skier work exceptionally hard. At the world-class level of competition in cross-country skiing, the heart is able to pump more blood than it does in any other sport or at any other time — some 25 quarts a minute, which is about six times the amount pumped by an untrained resting heart. Vigorous cross-country skiing also promotes large lung capacity, as well as the ability to take in air and expel it rapidly. The well-trained skier can process as much as seven quarts of air in less than three seconds.

For these reasons, cross-country skiers, along with runners, generally have the highest VO$_2$max values of any group of athletes. And one skier — Olympic gold medal-winner Sven-Åke Lundbäck of Sweden — has the highest VO$_2$max ever recorded.

Besides having well-developed aerobic capabilities, skiers tend to be well muscled. The leg motion of cross-country skiing conditions the calf and quadriceps particularly well, while poling conditions the triceps and the deltoid muscles in the arms and shoulders. Along with these muscles, skiing exercises muscle groups in the abdomen, chest and back — in all, more muscles than any other exercise. The fact that so many muscles are engaged also makes the energy costs of cross-country skiing high. Someone skiing continuously for two and a half hours may burn up nearly 3,000 calories.

Cross-country not only provides an excellent workout, but its smooth push-and-glide movement is virtually free of stress. Skiers sustain far fewer injuries than runners. According to one survey, only 49 injuries — half of them not serious — occurred among skiers skiing a total of 59,000 days over two years. Most of these were injuries due to falls or collisions on a downhill portion of a course, rather than stress injuries from overworked muscles.

Not least of all, cross-country skiing is fun, combining the pleasures of skiing and hiking. A good cross-country skier can cover five to 15 miles in a day of touring, and the variety of places to ski and explore is limitless. Skiers can either blaze their own trails or follow manicured ski trails with prepared tracks. (At least 35 states, including Hawaii, offer ski trails.) Furthermore, the equipment for cross-country is both lighter and less expensive than that for downhill.

Along with these advantages, cross-country skiing has the singular disadvantage of being a seasonal activity dependent on snow covering. Therefore, to maintain your aerobic fitness year-round, you have to take up such other activities as biking or running during the off-season. You can choose any one of the other endurance activities to maintain your basic aerobic fitness, but to stay in shape specifically for cross-country skiing, you must continue in an exercise similar to skiing. The traditional choice for skiers has been running. But many skiing coaches now recommend cycling, since cyclists' injury rate is lower than runners' and cycling conditions many of the same muscle groups as skiing. Race walking is another good off-season conditioner. Competitive cross-country skiers also frequently maintain their off-season fitness by walking or running with poles and skating on roller skis or skate blades.

You do not have to bundle up for cross-country as you would for downhill skiing, since your body generates plenty of extra heat. Also, heavy clothing interferes with the flexibility you need for arm swings and leg kicks. The traditional outfit of long underwear, sweater, knickers and knee socks is still acceptable. Racing skiers, however, frequently wear tight-fitting one-piece body suits, while the average fitness skier may choose what many winter runners prefer — layers of

Cross-Country Program Tips

◆ If you are a beginner, you can start by skiing without poles in ski tracks on "the flat," a term skiers use for a stretch of level ground. The exercise effort comes from taking a series of short steps, then gliding. This exercise will also teach you the importance of balance, weight shift and proper kicking. Once you can ski a good diagonal stride *(pages 104-105)*, you will get ever-increasing aerobic benefits by adding energy to your arm and leg movements, extending them and speeding them up.

◆ Adjust your tempo and technique to snow conditions. In dry, fast snow, you will move best with a short, powerful kick and a long glide. Wet snow pulls on the ski bottom, ruling out a long glide; therefore, shorten the slide but quicken the tempo of your stride to maintain the same energy expenditure as on dry snow.

◆ As you gain confidence in your ability, try skiing uphill using the diagonal stride. Choose a gradual incline with well-defined tracks. To work your heart and lungs without becoming exhausted, shorten your stride but increase your tempo, pushing more forcefully from each foot so that you conclude each kick with a little bounce. If you feel the skis starting to slip, try standing more upright. Bend less at the waist and take quick, jogging steps so that you will kick down, not backward. For steeper hills, use the herringbone *(page 110)* if the diagonal stride is ineffective.

◆ On slight downhills, do not coast: Double pole to keep your heart rate within the target zone. Relax in a tuck or standing position only when your speed picks up substantially. Similarly, do not let up on the flat, which may seem an easy way to rest after taking a hill. Resume a vigorous pace using a strong kick and full extension of the arms and legs.

◆ In the off-season, maintain fitness by running, walking or cycling in the hilly type of terrain that characterizes most cross-country ski trails. Try ski striding, a walking stride performed with ski poles to work your arms and help maintain your coordination for skiing. Take long, powerful steps like those in the diagonal stride *(pages 104-105)* and swing your arms holding the poles, as you would skiing on snow. You can increase the effort by ski striding uphill. To avoid blunting the tips of your poles, ski stride on grass.

fabrics that lift away perspiration from the skin surface, with a top layer of nylon or some other wind-breaking material. On very cold and windy days, you will need a wool cap, mittens and two pairs of socks — an inner pair of cotton and an outer pair of wool.

The movements of cross-country skiing are not difficult to learn; in fact, they are similar to walking. To learn the movements well, however, takes practice and probably a few lessons with a good instructor. Too often, beginners simply tramp across the snow without kicking, gliding or using the poles for anything other than balance, mistakenly equating walking on skis with skiing. One helpful tip for improving your technique is to imitate a good skier, stride for stride, following about a yard or so behind. You can emulate the power of his stride and get a good workout as well.

Diagonal
Stride

For cross-country skiing over flat terrain and up moderate inclines — where you are likely to do most of your skiing — the classic technique is the diagonal stride. Its kick-and-glide movements combine running and ice skating. You push down and back like a runner, but you glide like a skater. The workhorse of Nordic skiing, the diagonal stride provides power, yet it can also be relaxing.

In addition to the legs, the arms also supply force. The pole straps should be adjusted so that you can pull down on them, rather than having to grip the poles with your hands, which tires your hands and forearms unnecessarily. Pulling down, then pushing back, creates forward momentum. At the same time, your feet provide a strong push because the skis grip the snow as you step forward and kick back.

1

Start the stride by planting the pole in the snow, making sure that your hand is ahead of the pole tip for better leverage. Your body should be hunched slightly forward.

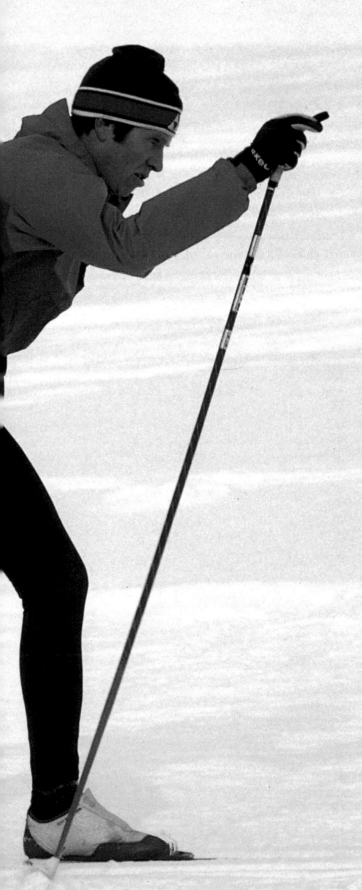

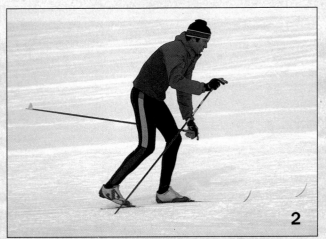

As you begin the kick with your left leg, concentrate on pressing the whole foot into the ski so that it can grip the snow. Push on the strap of the pole; do not grip the handle.

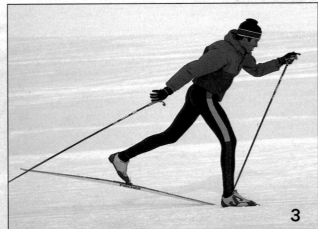

As you complete the kick, relax both your pushing arm and your propelling leg. Keep the front of your ski in contact with the snow at all times, even at the end of your kick.

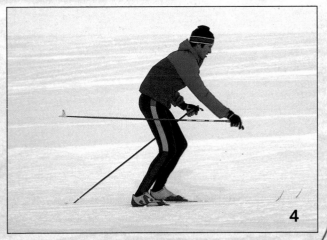

During the glide, both your recovering hand and the opposite foot swing forward in a relaxed, pendulum-like motion. Keep your knees bent and your body leaning forward.

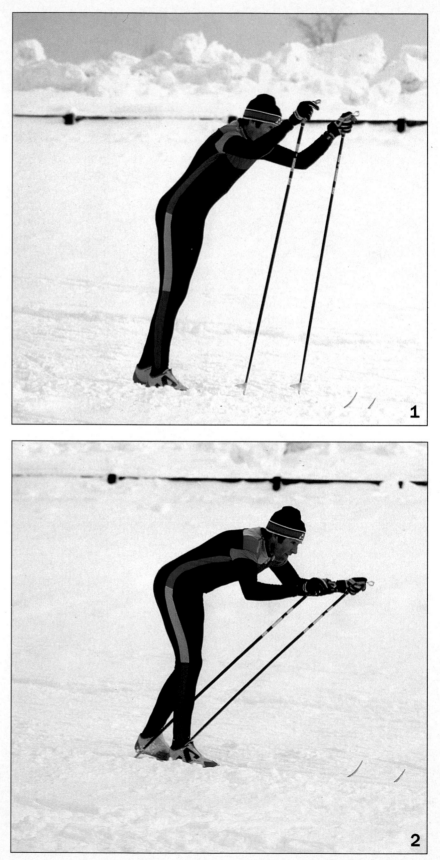

Rock forward to begin your push, and let one foot trail slightly behind the other for better balance. "Hang" on the straps so that your body weight gives you momentum.

When your feet reach the place where your poles are planted, flex at the waist and push to the rear. Keep looking forward throughout the push.

1

2

Double Poling

You can use double poling to work your arms, abdomen, back and shoulders, and to give your legs a rest after a long uphill climb. Double poling is most effective on level ground and is one of the fastest ways of skiing on gradual downhill slopes.

The technique is simple: You swing your arms forward with the poles to push down, then backward. With your elbows bent at about a 90-degree angle, keep your feet flat on the skis and plant your poles so that they are angled backward. Then, as your skis slide forward and your knees bend, pull down on the pole straps so that your body weight helps you move forward. Your shoulder muscles do the rest. Keep your elbows close to your body, since poling away from your line of travel at even a slight angle not only wastes energy but may throw you off balance.

As you slide farther forward, you bend over so that even your stomach muscles contribute to the push. Bending helps keep the poles in contact with the snow, giving you more time to apply pressure on them. Just as your poles are about to leave the snow, extend your wrists against the straps for one final push. The momentum carries your hands up past your hips so that they almost touch. Your knees stay slightly bent, but not flexed so much that your thigh muscles become excessively fatigued.

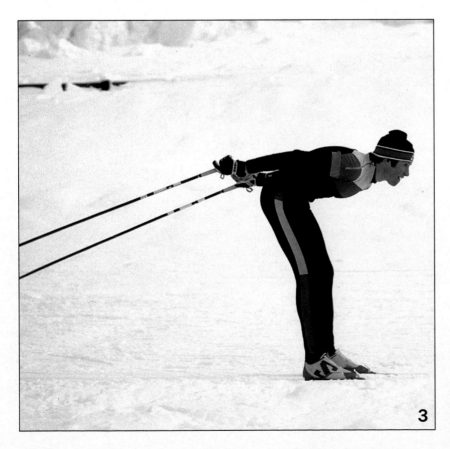

3

Extend the poles behind you. Bend at the waist, keeping your back flat, so that your arms and poles form a straight line almost horizontal to the ground.

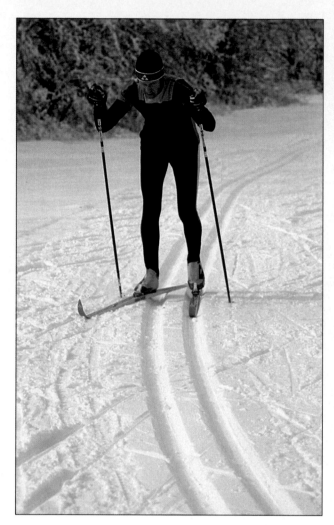

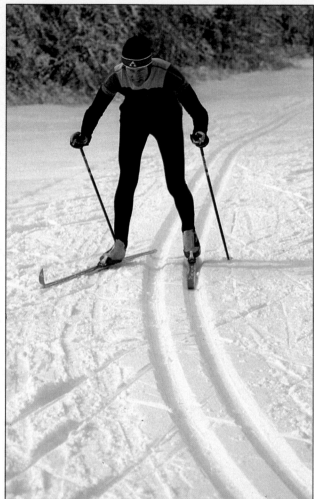

Skating

The fastest cross-country skiing stride is a relatively new technique called skating that was perfected by the U.S. Ski Team. It is also the most vigorous, since the skis are constantly in motion. The movement, which closely resembles ice skating, is used primarily for flat and gradual uphill terrain.

Technically called "the marathon skate" because it was developed by long-distance ski racers, the technique requires that you leave one ski in the track while pushing the other ski out to the side and simultaneously double poling. Angling one ski out of the track creates a small ledge for the ski to push against. The leg thrust, along with double poling, makes this stride both physically demanding and very fast.

While skating, you do not kick the skis backward, as in the diagonal stride. Skating involves a sideways push, much like an ice skater's stride, while the ski is still in motion. This may feel like an unnatural movement for beginning skiers.

Because marathon skating pushes one ski against and across the track, it can damage ski tracks. It is therefore prohibited on some trails. A variation on the marathon skate that can be done outside the track to preserve it is the double-pole V skate, shown on the opposite page.

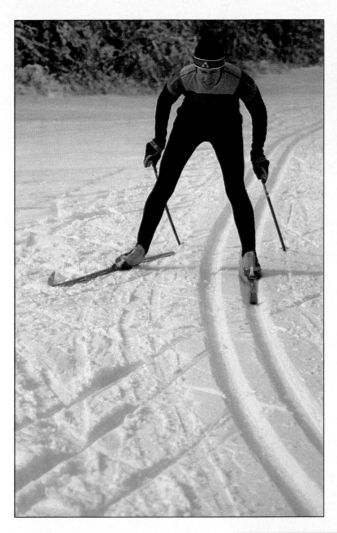

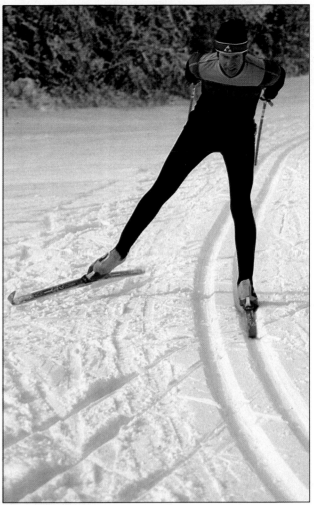

To begin the marathon skate *(opposite, far left)*, stand on both skis, one in the track, the other slanted to the side. Your heels should be even and the ski tails should cross each other. Double pole and lean toward the slanting ski to maintain balance while it moves away *(opposite, left)*. As the ski continues to move out *(above)*, turn it slightly on its inside edge so that it creates its own ledge for pushing off. As you push off, complete the double pole *(above right)*. Your skating foot should be about even with your other foot so that you return to the initial position without losing your balance. For skating over long distances, repeat this sequence four to seven times on one leg, then shift to the other leg.

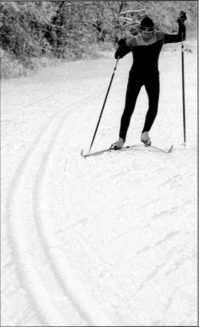

Start the double-pole V skate, which is done outside the track, much as you would the marathon skate. But angle the skis to form a V and use the gliding ski to perform an alternating skate without the double pole *(right)*.

109

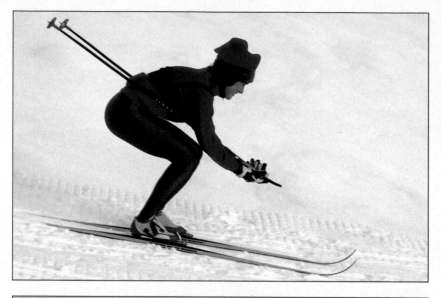

Downhill Technique

In order to maintain your target heart rate, you must keep moving and get through the "resting" phases of skiing as efficiently as possible. Going downhill, assume a relaxed, upright position with your knees and ankles slightly flexed and your hands down and forward. By employing a tuck position *(top left)*, you can increase your downhill speed and at the same time lower your center of gravity to improve stability. Tuck the poles under your arms as you assume a crouching stance, with the bulk of your weight toward the tails of your skis. To decrease your speed on a downhill, press your pole tips down behind you, dragging them over the snow. You can also snowplow, or wedge *(middle left)*. Make an A with your skis, bending your knees and moving the tips of the skis together while moving the tails apart. The wider the A, the greater the braking power.

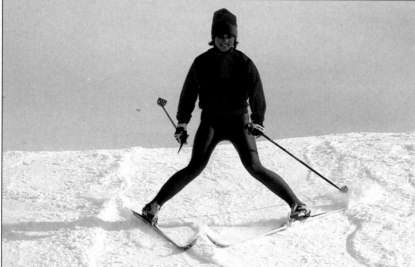

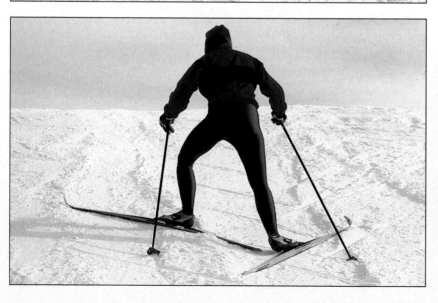

Uphill Technique

One effective method for getting up steep slopes is virtually the reverse of the wedge — the herringbone. Form a V with your skis, and keep your poles at your sides and outside the skis *(left)*. Put your weight on the inside edge of the skis so that a small ledge of snow forms on each step to push off from. Bend your knees and lift your skis over each other so that they pass close together without touching. Keep your head up, your eyes ahead and your buttocks tucked in; otherwise, you may lean over your skis and cause them to lose traction.

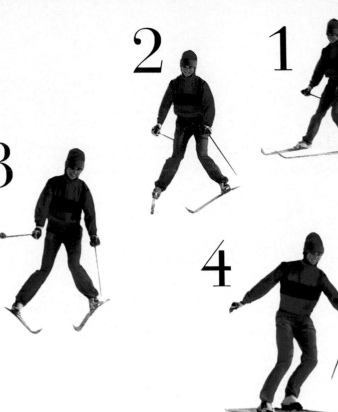

Wedge Turn

You can use the wedge on a downhill not only for braking, but also for turning. To execute a left turn, form a narrow A with your skis (1) and use the outside right foot to steer. Transfer your weight to the right ski (2) while turning your toe in and pushing your heel out (3). Finally, bring your left ski parallel to your right (4).

Telemark Turn

This technique is most effective in powder snow, though it is easier to learn on a packed surface. Make a left turn by transferring your weight to your left ski (1). Slide the right ski ahead of the left until the binding of the right ski is near the tip of the left (2). The lower your body position and the farther apart your feet, the greater your stability and control. To make the turn, put your weight on the inside ski. As you come around the turn (3), balance your weight equally on both skis (4). Complete the turn by assuming an upright position again (5). Bring your left foot forward until it is even with the right.

Equipment

Cross-country skis must perform two opposing functions — grip the snow and glide across it. To accomplish this, the skis are constructed with a bow-like camber, or arch. The gripping part of the ski is in the center and the gliding portions at the ends. When the skier applies enough pressure, the ski flattens against the snow.

Generally, your skis have the right camber if a friend can slip a piece of paper between your skis and a hard, smooth floor while you are standing in them. When you balance your weight on one ski, the paper should be clamped to the floor.

There are two basic types of cross-country skis: waxless and waxable. Waxless skis have patterns along their bottoms that grip the snow, while waxable skis require applications of various types of wax. Waxless skis are slower than the waxables and cannot be used for skating. However, many noncompetitive skiers prefer them because they require less care and generally hold better on the uphills.

Boots of leather or synthetic materials are clamped to the ski at the toe. This gives you maximum flexibility while still allowing you control over the ski.

The "hairy," a ski bottom with a strip of short silicon-coated fiberglass hairs, is the best waxless ski on new snow when the temperature hovers around freezing.

The fish-scale pattern is a popular waxless bottom design. Reliable and strong on uphills, it can slip on hard or icy tracks.

A scalloped or shingled pattern like this is also popular. Generally, the greater the number of angles, the better the hold, but a "stamped-in" pattern does not grip snow as well as a raised one.

For most techniques, the pole should be at least as high as your armpit. For skating, the pole should reach your chin or higher.

n Italy

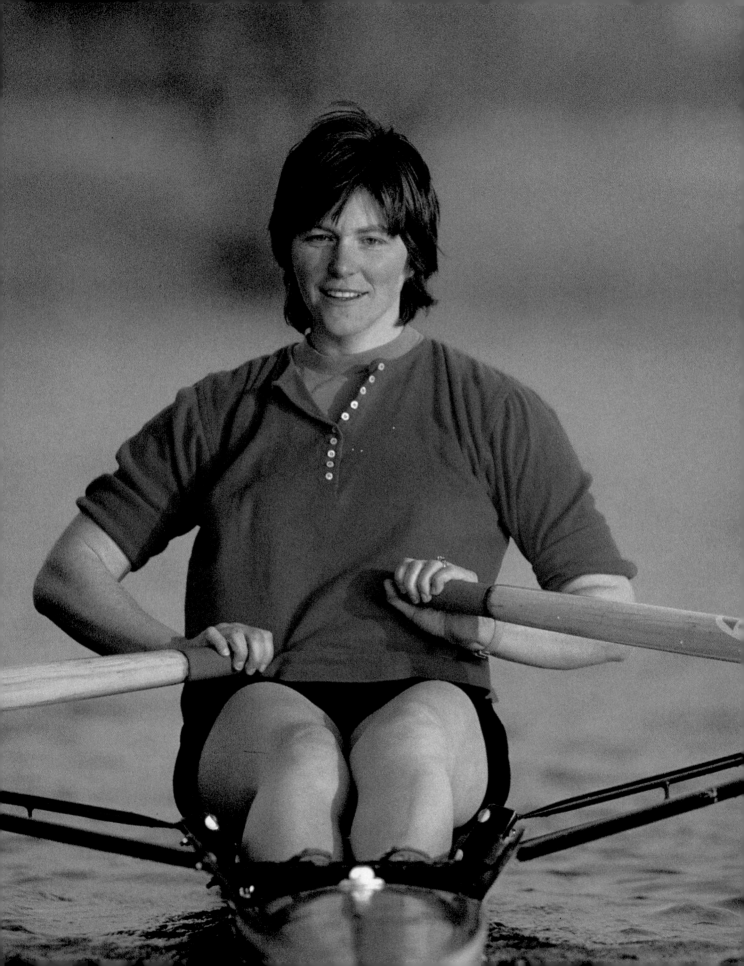

CHAPTER EIGHT

Rowing

*Once the exclusive sport
of the Ivy League, now the ultimate
fair-weather workout
for the serious fitness enthusiast*

More than any other exercise, rowing combines the benefits of endurance and strength. Rowers use their upper bodies to take powerful strokes with oars, and they can intensify the stroking motion by sliding back and forth with their legs in seats that roll on tracks. Whether you are stroking on the water in a shell or on land using a machine that mimics the operation of a shell, regular rowing provides considerable rewards.

Because rowing uses muscles in the arms, legs, abdomen, torso and the buttocks, rowers tend to be lean and well developed, yet not immensely muscular (except perhaps in the thighs and upper back). The well-conditioned rower is bound to be superbly fit aerobically; top rowers can consume almost seven quarts of oxygen per minute, an amount greater than that consumed by elite runners or even cross-country skiers. The energy output of rowers is equally impressive: about 36 calories per minute as compared with 30 for cross-country skiers. Rowing a shell also develops coordination. An added dividend is the sense of relaxation that comes from smoothly propelling oneself through the water. Finally, all of these direct benefits may contribute to increased longevity: A study of Ivy League varsity oarsmen revealed that rowers outlived their nonrowing classmates by an average of six years.

What makes these benefits possible — and has also broadened rowing's appeal — is the modern rowing shell, a lightweight, streamlined vessel that can skim across water at speeds up to eight mph, far faster than a plain rowboat. And unlike a rowboat, the shell has a sliding seat that turns it into a full-body exercising apparatus. By sliding back and forth in the seat, you drive a shell not only with your arm and back muscles, but with your abdomen, thighs and calves as well.

In fact, although your arms directly drive the oars, it is the large muscles of the thighs that provide most of your power. The quadriceps muscles along the front of the thighs extend the legs during the propulsive, or drive, phase of the stroke when you pull the boat through the water. After you lift the oar blades out of the water, the hamstring muscles in the back of the thighs draw the knees up to move the seat forward and return the rower to his starting position.

Because the quadriceps and hamstrings constantly work in alternation, rowers have about the strongest thigh muscles of all athletes. Biopsies of the leg muscles of elite rowers show they have a significantly higher than average percentage of slow-twitch fibers, the type of muscle fiber that most effectively uses oxygen during aerobic activity.

Despite the heavy demands it places on the body, rowing is a relatively stress-free exercise that has a low injury rate. A study of more than 2,000 rowers indicates that the joint and muscle problems that afflict runners are not evident among people who row regularly. One of the few annoyances are blisters, which can be avoided by taping the hands. Rowing so effectively strengthens back muscles that sports physicians sometimes prescribe it for people with lower back and disk problems. (For some types of back conditions, however, rowing is not a suitable exercise. If you have back trouble, check with your physician. People with heart trouble should also approach rowing with caution, since it accelerates the heart rate rapidly.)

In recent years, rowing has become more accessible. This is largely due to the development of easy-to-handle fiberglass boats that are stable enough to be used in coastal waters as well as in the calmer waters of lakes and rivers. Furthermore, a growing number of communities and universities provide public access to rowing facilities, and many rowing clubs offer programs for beginners.

Although it has broken away from its image as an elite sport of the Ivy League, rowing is still a relatively expensive exercise. A good recreational rowing shell and oars cost more than $1,500. And once you have a shell, you will need a shed or boathouse to store it and a trailer or automobile roof rack to transport it.

Another drawback is that rowing is seasonal and dependent on the weather and water conditions. If you do not live in a mild climate year-round, you must take up another endurance activity to maintain

Rowing Program Tips

◆ Whether you use a shell or a rowing machine, begin your workouts with a progressive slide — a routine in which you move farther along on the sliding seat with each set of strokes. With the seat all the way back at the finish position, row 20 strokes only with your arms; 20 strokes with your arms and back using a quarter of the slide on each stroke; then 20 strokes using three quarters of the slide; and finally 20 strokes using the full slide. This establishes your rhythm and balance and warms up the right muscles. Moreover, rowing without using the slide is the best way to learn handling the oars.

◆ For the first few weeks of your rowing program, gradually increase the pressure you exert on the oar to what rowers call three quarters, which is 75 percent of what you could do if you had to work as hard as possible. You will be pushing yourself but not so hard that you run out of breath.

◆ As you become more fit, add speed training to your workouts. You can divide your workout into sequences of rowing at different pressures (the amount of force you apply to the oar). Begin with five minutes of paddling, in which you put only light pressure on the oars. Follow with five minutes at half your maximum pressure, then two minutes at three-quarter pressure, building up to a minute at full pressure to bring you to peak exertion. Then reverse the sequence, going back down to five minutes at half pressure and finishing with five minutes of paddling.

◆ Many rowers train by doing power pieces, a set number of strokes at full pressure. You can arrange the power pieces into pyramids. For example, row a power-10, which is 10 strokes at full pressure, then 10 easy strokes. Other variations you can try are a power-20, then 10 easy strokes; a power-30, then 15 easy, 40 then 20, 50 then 30 and back down to a power-10. Because power pieces bring short-term anaerobic energy sources into play, you should alternate power-piece workouts with workouts of longer pieces at steady power.

◆ As your rowing style improves, experiment with your stroke rating, which is the number of strokes you take per minute. Regardless of the pressure you are using, the stroke-to-recovery ratio should never be less than 1 to 1. That means your oars should never spend more time in the water than out of the water. One way to build up strength is to alternate stroke ratings. Try a slow rating of 18 strokes per minute on one of your power pieces. Then try 30. This exercise will improve your glide and, with that, your speed. In a recreational shell, you will find that 20 to 22 strokes per minute is a solid rating for your workouts.

your aerobic fitness. During the winter, many rowers run, cross-country ski and work out on rowing machines (see box page 116).

Since most rowers take an occasional spill, it is essential that you know how to swim and carry on board a life jacket or personal flotation device. While rowing, wear clothing appropriate for the weather. Because your body will generate a lot of heat, do not overdress.

Most people who row for fitness prefer the convenience of a single scull, a shell for one rower. Most single recreational shells are built for moderate-paced, long-distance cruising. They are maneuverable in choppy water, and their fiberglass hulls are sturdy and can be beached on the sand without damage if you want to get out and explore.

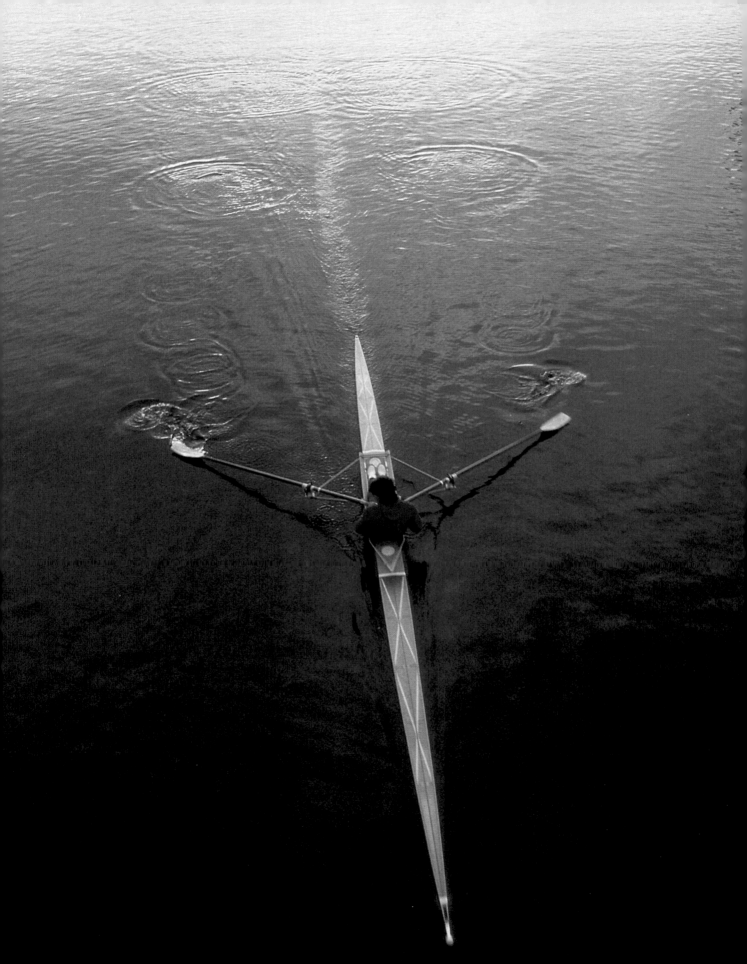

Balance and Stroke

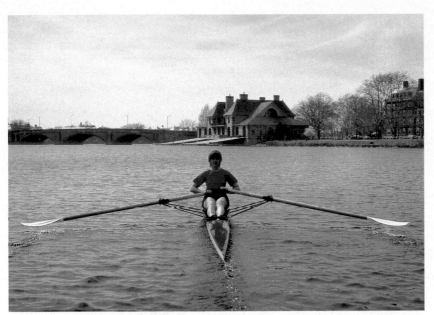

To balance a shell, center your body precisely *(above)*. Keep your hands at about the same height and your knees together at all times. Make sure that the starboard oarlock is half an inch higher than the one at port so that the left oarhandle will pass over the right one.

When you are rowing, watch the puddles left by your oar. The farther apart they are, the better you are gliding — the key to an efficient stroke. The rower at left has just finished a stroke, leaving a puddle by each oar. The previous stroke ended at the large puddles several yards beyond the stern.

The first step in mastering a rowing shell is keeping your balance, whether you are in a racing shell like the models here or in a recreational shell such as the one on pages 122-123. Center your weight and make sure that the oars are level with one another throughout the stroke. And never let go of an oar. A full stroke cycle consists of two phases: the drive through the water and the recovery *(pages 120-121)*. For the drive, you "catch" the water with your oar, push off with your legs, then finish with your back and arms to propel the shell into a fast, smooth glide. You then release the oar from the water and recover.

During the recovery, your weight slides toward the stern, contributing acceleration to the boat. Most beginners rush to the next stroke by rolling back on the sliding seat too quickly, checking the boat's glide. The recovery should be longer than the time the oar is in the water.

Throughout the stroke, strive for a relaxed body. You should feel strong but not tense during the drive. Let your legs do all the early work, while your back and arms merely transfer the pressure to the oar. Then slowly swing your torso toward the bow. Never jerk backward or use your back muscles for the bulk of the power. This can cause injury.

Handling the oars takes practice. During the drive, the blades of the oars are squared, or perpendicular to the water surface. During the recovery, try to feather the oars — turn the blades almost parallel to the water — so they move easily through the air back to the drive position. It is helpful to practice this one hand at a time without sliding on the seat, while someone holds the bow of the shell.

119

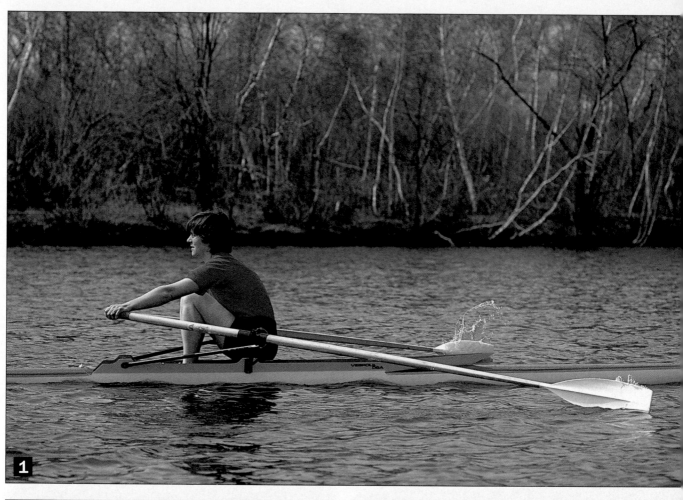

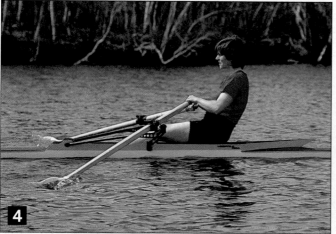

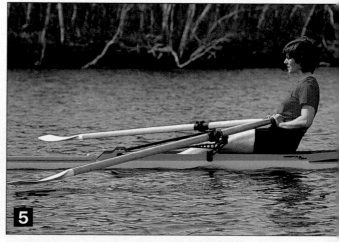

4. Continue working your back. Just after you pass the upright position, pull your arms quickly to your body for the finish. Keep the blade in the water to the end.

5. Release the oars from the water by moving the handles down with your forearms while your legs and back remain in the finish position. Cock your wrists to feather the oars.

Stroking
Step by Step

1. At the catch, roll forward on your sliding seat until your shins are vertical. Reach with your arms and shoulders. Raise only the hands to drop the blades into the water quickly and cleanly. Then begin the leg drive. Keep your wrists straight, with thumbs exerting slight outward pressure on the end of the oarhandle. Your head should be upright throughout the stroke sequence, and you should breathe evenly.

2. During the early part of the drive, your legs do the work. Do not change body position. Feel your back transmit the power of your legs as you drive your weight toward the bow.

3. Gradually let your back muscles take over as your legs extend and your body uncoils. Pass your starboard oarhandle over the port handle in midstroke.

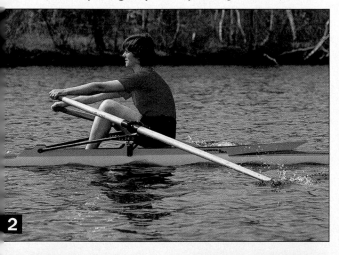

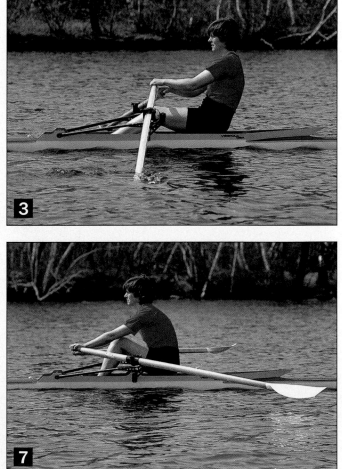

6. Move your hands away from your body at a steady speed and follow with your shoulders. Begin rolling up the slide once your hands have passed your knees.

7. To prepare for the catch, square the blades as your hands pass your ankles. Continue rolling up the slide until your shins are vertical.

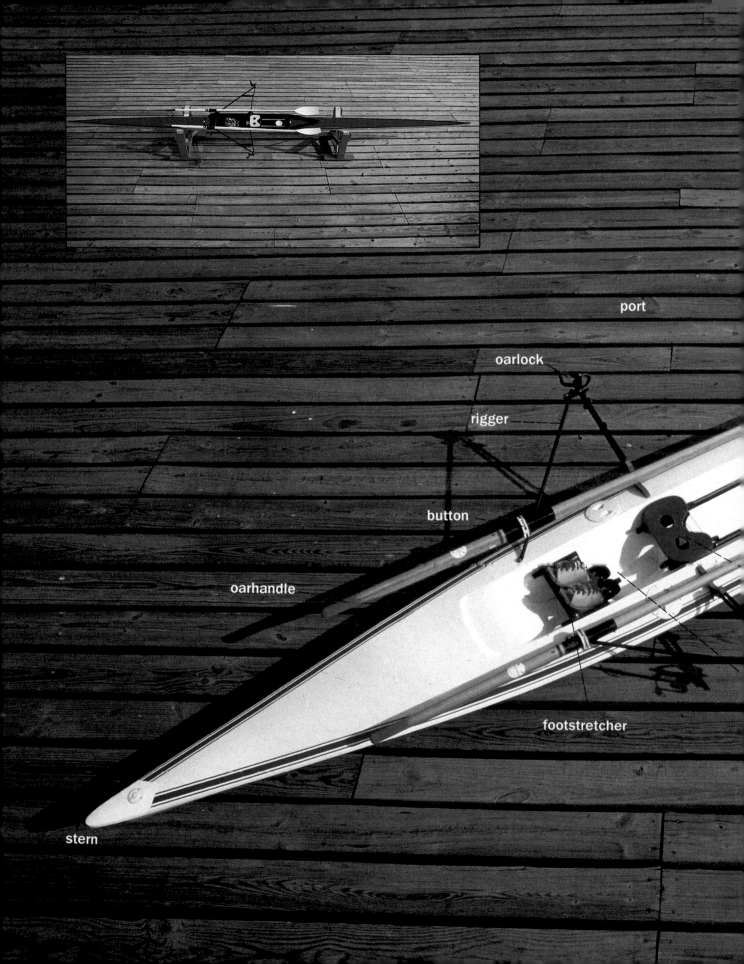

port

oarlock

rigger

button

oarhandle

footstretcher

stern

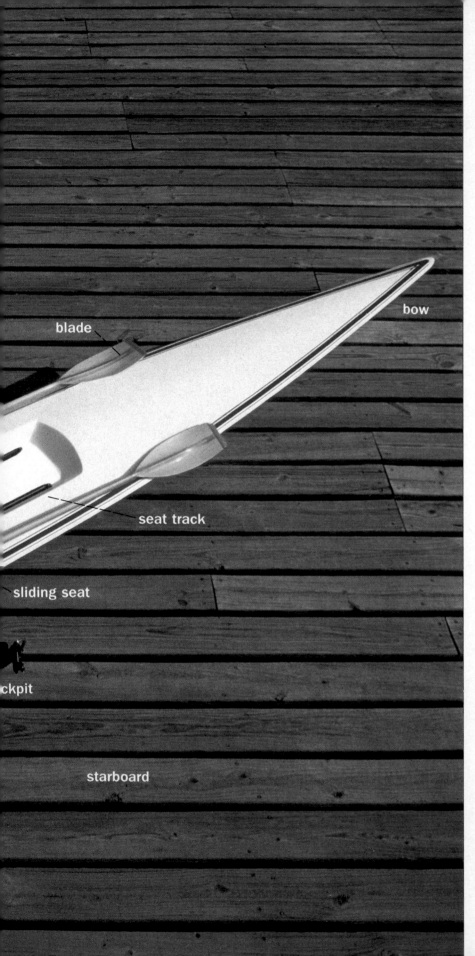

blade

bow

seat track

sliding seat

ckpit

starboard

Using a Rowing Shell

You can row in either a racing shell or a recreational shell; both work the same way. However, a recreational shell such as the one at left is fairly wide and therefore more stable than a racing shell. This makes the recreational shell not only easier to balance, but also suitable for rougher water, which can capsize racing shells.

Rowing shells are equipped with adjustable parts. Before going out on any row, check that all nuts and bolts on the riggers are tight, and install the seat on the tracks. When you get into the shell, adjust the position of the footstretcher. It is set correctly when, as you sit in the finish position holding the oars, your thumbs just touch the bottom of your rib cage. Other adjustments you can make, if necessary, are the height and pitch of the oarlocks and their distance from the side of the boat.

The moving parts of the boat that are vulnerable to damage by friction and dirt — the button of the oar (which holds the oar in the oarlock), the oarlock, the rollers on the seat — should be kept clean and greased.

Use a footstretcher that allows your feet to slide out. You can row as well and more safely than with attached shoes.

The adjustments above also apply to racing shells, the preferred equipment of many experienced rowers. Narrower than recreational shells and difficult to balance, racing shells are designed for speed on a straight course under ideal conditions. Try a racing shell only after you have mastered a recreational shell.

The width of recreational shells gives them stability. The model at left is 26 inches wide as compared with the 11-inch width of the racing shell *(inset)*. The parts on a recreational shell are also sturdier and easier to care for.

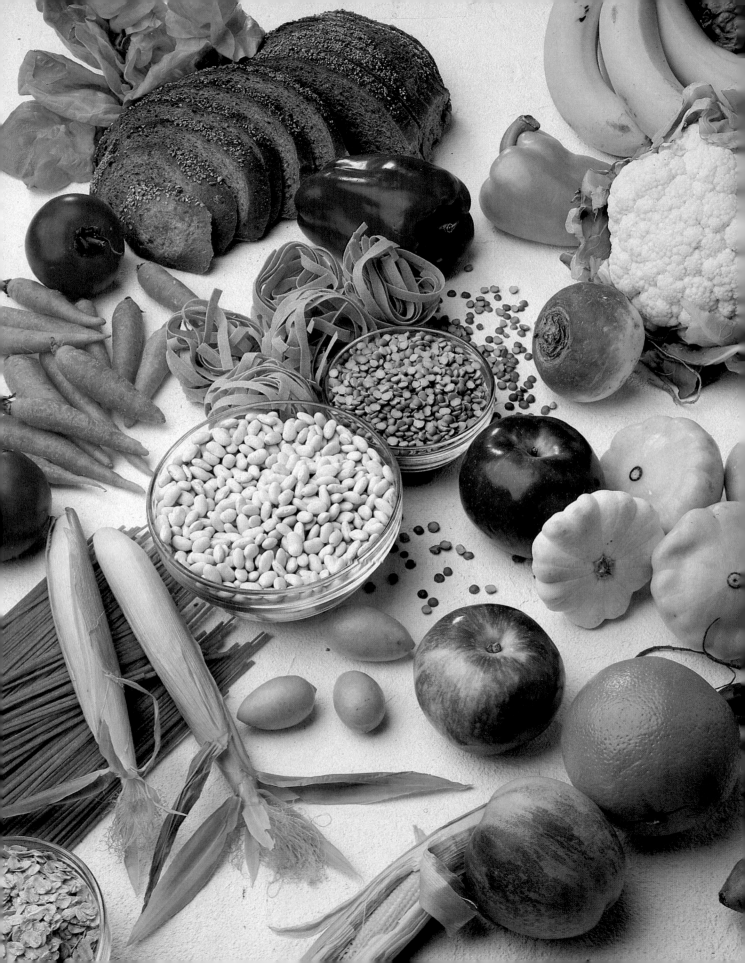

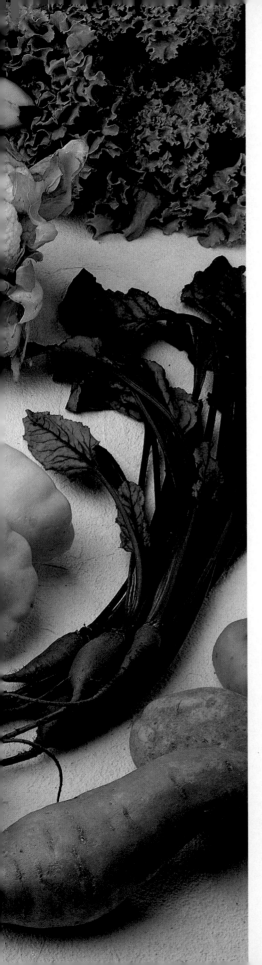

CHAPTER NINE

Carbohydrates

The primary fuel for endurance

No single food or food group provides the magic road to health or fitness. But foods rich in carbohydrates — cereals and grains, fruits and vegetables — supply our chief source of energy. Even at a moderate level of activity, we draw on carbohydrates for 50 percent or more of our energy needs. As our activity becomes more intense, so does carbohydrate use: Someone running at 75 percent of his capacity, for example, is fueled almost entirely by carbohydrates. And studies confirm that athletes on a high-carbohydrate diet have three times the endurance of athletes on a diet high in fat, the other principal energy fuel.

Whatever your level of physical activity, carbohydrates can go a long way toward enhancing your endurance. The key is choosing the right kind of carbohydrates and replenishing them daily. Whereas the body can store an almost unlimited amount of fat from excess food consumption, it can retain only a limited supply of carbohydrates, at most about 1,500 calories. If you fast for a day and sustain a normal level of activity at the same time, you will deplete most of those carbohydrates.

Carbohydrates come in two types — simple and complex. The simple carbohydrates are the sugars. They include glucose and fructose from fruits and vegetables, lactose from milk, and sucrose from cane or beet sugar. Whether refined or unrefined, most sugars are broken down in the small intestine during digestion. Eventually they travel to the liver and from there to the bloodstream as glucose. The cells use some of this glucose for immediate energy and store some for future use. The surplus may end up in the liver and muscles as glycogen, which can also be converted to glucose for energy.

Complex carbohydrates, which are large chains of simple sugars, are found mainly in the starches in potatoes, beans, cereal and grains, and the cellulose of fiber that occurs in the bran, or outer shell, of grains and in other plant foods. Foods that contain complex carbohydrates may contain some simple ones as well.

A critical difference, however, between a starchy potato and a sugar-packed chocolate bar is that the high concentration of the sugar in the candy provides too much too soon. It raises the blood's glucose level, but the body responds by releasing insulin, the hormone that enables glucose to enter the cells. Almost immediately, the glucose drops to a level even lower than it was before the candy was eaten. The body then has to call prematurely upon glycogen reserves in the muscles, causing the muscles to tire faster than they normally would.

Another reason for choosing complex over simple carbohydrates is to avoid unwanted body fat. The glucose from sugar-rich foods is so much more than the body can use at any one time that a large share of it is converted to fat. In addition, the various forms of sugar in sweets make up such a large proportion of the calories that the sugars crowd out protein and other critical nutrients.

Foods rich in complex carbohydrates can also pack plenty of calories, but the nutrients that the package includes more than compensate for them. Two slices of whole-wheat bread, for example, may contain 130 calories, nearly the same as a soft drink, which may have 150 calories. The bread gives you some protein, a small amount of fat, B vitamins, calcium and iron, as well as fiber; most soft drinks offer none of these. Because starches are digested more slowly than simple sugars, they also fill us up in a satisfying way. And far from causing the insulin reaction that sugar does, complex carbohydrates release a slower but steady supply of glucose into the system over a long period of time.

Realizing that carbohydrates supply the energy they need, endurance athletes such as marathon runners have tried to boost their performance by increasing their intake of carbohydrates. A number of studies indicate that a diet in which carbohydrates make up 70 percent or more of the total calories can increase the glycogen stored in the muscles. This, in turn, helps stave off fatigue. Some athletes go one step further for three to four days before an endurance event by "carbo loading," eating foods that are 70 to 80 percent carbohydrates.

Not all researchers accept the validity of carbohydrate loading.

The Basic Guidelines

For a moderately active adult, the National Institutes of Health recommends a diet that is low in fat, high in carbohydrates and moderate in protein. The institutes' guidelines suggest that no more than 30 percent of your calories come from fat, that 55 to 60 percent come from carbohydrates and that no more than 15 percent come from protein. A gram of fat equals nine calories, while a gram of protein or carbohydrate equals four calories; therefore, if you eat 2,100 calories a day, you should consume approximately 60 grams of fat, 315 grams of carbohydrate and no more than 75 grams of protein daily. If you follow a lowfat/high-carbohydrate diet, your chance of developing heart disease, cancer and other life-threatening diseases may be considerably reduced.

The nutrition charts that accompany each of the lowfat/high-carbohydrate recipes in this book include the number of calories per serving, the number of grams of fat, carbohydrate and protein in a serving, and the percentage of calories derived from each of these nutrients. In addition, the charts provide the amount of calcium, iron and sodium per serving.

Calcium deficiency may be associated with periodontal disease — which attacks the mouth's bones and tissues, including the gums — in both men and women, and with osteoporosis, or bone shrinking and weakening, in the elderly. The deficiency may also contribute to high blood pressure. The recommended daily allowance for calcium is 800 milligrams a day for men and women. Pregnant and lactating women are advised to consume 1,200 milligrams daily; a National Institutes of Health consensus panel recommends that postmenopausal women consume 1,200 to 1,500 milligrams of calcium daily.

Although one way you can reduce your fat intake is to cut your consumption of red meat, you should make sure that you get your necessary iron from other sources. The Food and Nutrition Board of the National Academy of Sciences suggests a minimum of 10 milligrams of iron per day for men and 18 milligrams for women between the ages of 11 and 50.

High sodium intake is associated with high blood pressure. Most adults should restrict sodium intake to between 2,000 and 2,500 milligrams a day, according to the National Academy of Sciences. One way to keep sodium consumption in check is not to add table salt to food.

Those who do accept it, however, agree that any benefits from a high-carbohydrate regimen apply only to bouts of exercise lasting at least one and a half to two hours, when normal stores of glycogen become exhausted. So for anyone not competing in the top ranks of marathons, triathlons or other endurance contests, special diets are clearly unnecessary — and, by throwing an ordinarily healthy diet out of whack, such diets may do some harm.

The best way, in fact, to enhance your exercise program and maximize endurance is to eat a balanced diet. Most nutritionists suggest that you get 55 percent to 60 percent of your calories from carbohydrates, primarily complex carbohydrates. The recipes that follow provide at least this proportion, and some are more than 70 percent carbohydrates. By themselves, these dishes do not constitute a balanced diet. But if you feel that you have been stinting on carbohydrates, you may want to incorporate some of these recipes into your diet.

Breakfast

· · · · · · · · · · · · · · · · · · · ·

CALORIES	342
78% Carbohydrate	66 g
12% Protein	10 g
10% Fat	4 g
CALCIUM	117 mg
IRON	3 mg
SODIUM	453 mg

The nutritional analyses accompanying these recipes provide nutrient values per serving, unless otherwise indicated.

ORANGE-NUTMEG PAN TOAST

Eating this carbohydrate-rich dish right after your morning workout, when your muscles store glycogen most efficiently, will help boost your energy level for the rest of the day.

1 egg

1/2 cup skim milk

1 teaspoon grated orange peel

1/4 teaspoon nutmeg

8 slices whole-wheat French bread, 1/2 inch thick

1/2 cup maple syrup

1 tablespoon confectioners' sugar

Place the egg, milk, 2 tablespoons of water, the orange peel and nutmeg in a large shallow pan, and whisk to combine. Place the bread slices in the egg mixture to coat one side, then immediately turn the bread. Let the bread stand at least 10 minutes. Warm the syrup in a small saucepan. Preheat a nonstick griddle or a large nonstick skillet over medium heat. Brown both sides of the bread slices on the griddle or in the skillet. Sprinkle with sugar and serve with warm syrup.   4 servings

Orange-Nutmeg Pan Toast

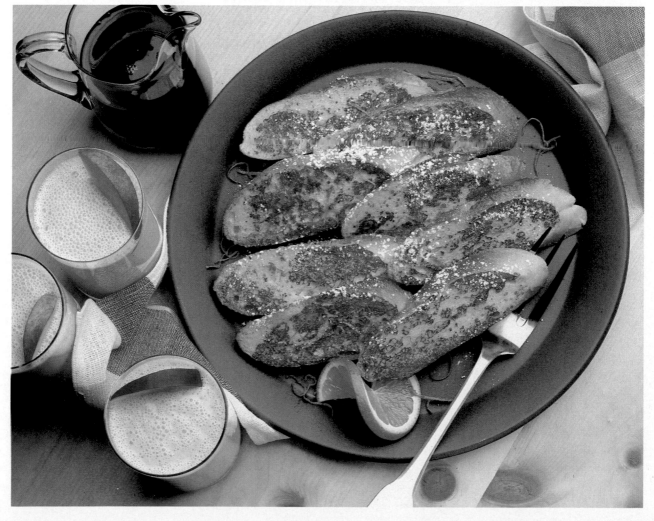

JAM MUFFINS

*High in complex carbohydrates, whole-wheat muffins are among the
pre-race favorites of competitive cyclists.*

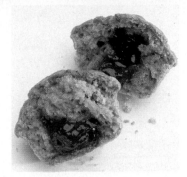

2 cups whole-wheat flour	1/4 cup honey
2 teaspoons baking powder	1 teaspoon grated lemon or orange
1/4 teaspoon salt	peel
1 1/4 cups lowfat milk (1% fat)	2 tablespoons strawberry, raspberry or
1 egg, beaten	apricot jam
1/4 cup vegetable oil	2 tablespoons wheat germ

Preheat the oven to 400° F. Line 12 muffin pan cups with paper liners. In a
large bowl, mix the flour, baking powder and salt. Combine the milk, egg, oil,
honey and peel, and add to the flour mixture. Stir just until the dry ingredients
are moistened. Fill the muffin cups 1/4 full of batter. Spoon 1/2 teaspoon of
jam into each cup and top equally with the remaining batter. Sprinkle the batter
with wheat germ. Bake the muffins on the middle oven rack for 20 minutes, or
until browned on top and firm to the touch.   Makes 12 muffins

CALORIES per muffin	177
60% Carbohydrate	27 g
10% Protein	4 g
30% Fat	6 g
CALCIUM	56 mg
IRON	1 mg
SODIUM	132 mg

WAKE-UP SHAKE

*After exercise, the fresh fruit in this drink helps replace the minerals you lose
from sweating.*

1 nectarine, quartered and pitted	2 tablespoons wheat germ
1 cup plain lowfat yogurt	2 ice cubes
1/4 cup orange juice	

Place all the ingredients in a blender. Blend until well mixed, thick and frothy.
          1 serving

CALORIES	296
60% Carbohydrate	44 g
23% Protein	17 g
17% Fat	6 g
CALCIUM	432 mg
IRON	2 mg
SODIUM	161 mg

BUTTERMILK CORNMEAL PANCAKES

*Buttermilk, a lowfat milk product, is more easily digested than whole milk.
Buttermilk at breakfast is less likely to cause stomach cramps than the
slowly absorbed fat in whole milk.*

1 cup stone-ground yellow	1/4 teaspoon salt
cornmeal	1 egg
1/2 cup unbleached flour	1 1/4 cups buttermilk, approximately
1 tablespoon baking powder	1 tablespoon safflower oil
1/2 teaspoon baking soda	

Combine the dry ingredients in a large bowl. Add the egg, buttermilk and oil,
and stir to mix thoroughly. If the batter is too thick, add additional buttermilk by
the tablespoon. Preheat a nonstick griddle or a large nonstick skillet. Using a
scant 1/4 cup batter for each pancake, pour the batter onto the hot griddle or
into the skillet. Cook until bubbles just begin to form on the tops of the pancakes and the bottoms are lightly browned. Turn and cook the other side until
lightly browned.   Makes 12 pancakes (4 servings)

CALORIES	265
66% Carbohydrate	44 g
13% Protein	9 g
21% Fat	6 g
CALCIUM	160 mg
IRON	2 mg
SODIUM	641 mg

Lunch

. . . .

BAKED POTATOES WITH RATATOUILLE

CALORIES	297
66% Carbohydrate	49 g
10% Protein	8 g
24% Fat	8 g
CALCIUM	78 mg
IRON	3 mg
SODIUM	150 mg

Potatoes supply more vitamins and minerals than any other high-carbohydrate vegetable. Top triathletes — who train at running, swimming and cycling — sometimes eat eight or more a day.

4 baking potatoes
1 medium onion, sliced
1 medium eggplant, diced
1 medium zucchini, diced
1 medium yellow squash, diced
1 small green bell pepper, diced
1 small red bell pepper, diced

15-ounce can whole peeled tomatoes, with liquid
1 garlic clove, crushed
1/2 teaspoon dried oregano, crumbled
1/4 teaspoon red pepper flakes
2 tablespoons chopped fresh parsley

Preheat the oven to 350° F. Scrub and dry the potatoes and prick the skins a few times with a fork. Bake the potatoes for about 1 hour, or until easily pierced with a fork. Meanwhile, combine all the remaining ingredients except the parsley in a large nonstick skillet. Sauté over medium-high heat, breaking up the tomatoes with a spoon, for about 8 minutes, or until the vegetables begin to soften. Cover the skillet, reduce the heat to low and simmer for another 20 minutes. Halve the baked potatoes lengthwise without cutting through the bottom skin. Separate the halves and top each potato with ratatouille. Sprinkle with chopped parsley.   4 servings

LEEK AND POTATO SOUP

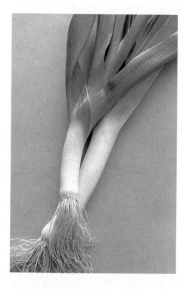

Unlike most canned soups, this homemade soup is low in sodium and fat.

4 to 5 leeks (about 1 pound)
2 potatoes, peeled and quartered
1 cup thinly sliced celery
4 cups low-sodium chicken stock

2 cups skim milk
1 tablespoon chopped fresh parsley
White pepper

CALORIES	218
67% Carbohydrate	37 g
24% Protein	13 g
9% Fat	2 g
CALCIUM	275 mg
IRON	4 mg
SODIUM	213 mg

Cut off the root ends and green tops from the leeks. Halve the leeks lengthwise, separate the layers and wash them thoroughly. Cut the leeks into 1-inch pieces. In a large saucepan, combine the leeks, potatoes, celery and stock. Bring to a boil, skimming off any scum. Reduce the heat and simmer, uncovered, for about 40 minutes, or until the vegetables are tender.

Cool the soup briefly, then purée in a blender or food processor or mash to a coarse purée by hand. Add the milk, and reheat the soup just until heated through; do not boil. Ladle the soup into bowls or mugs, and sprinkle with parsley and pepper.   4 servings

Orzo and Vegetables

ORZO AND VEGETABLES

Because pasta releases a slow, steady stream of glucose into the bloodstream, it makes a superb endurance fuel. Runners traditionally load up on pasta the night before a marathon.

2 cups orzo (rice-shaped pasta)
1 tablespoon vegetable oil
1/3 cup chopped onion
2 medium zucchini, cut into
  2" × 1/2" pieces

1 cup fresh or frozen corn kernels
1/4 cup chopped pecans
1 tablespoon chopped fresh dill

Cook the orzo according to package directions until al dente. Turn the orzo into a colander and set aside to drain. Meanwhile, heat the oil in a large skillet. Add the onion and sauté until transparent. Add the zucchini, corn and 1/4 cup water to the skillet, cover and cook the vegetables over medium heat for about 5 minutes, or until just tender. Add the orzo, pecans and dill to the skillet and cook, stirring, until heated through.
Note: This dish is also good served cold.

4 servings

CALORIES	313
62% Carbohydrate	49 g
11% Protein	9 g
27% Fat	10 g
CALCIUM	55 mg
IRON	2 mg
SODIUM	3 mg

LAMB IN PITA BREAD

The chickpeas in this recipe provide cholesterol-lowering fiber as well as extra carbohydrates and protein.

Eight 6-inch whole-wheat pitas
1/2 pound lean ground lamb
1/4 cup chopped onion
1/2 cup chopped green bell
  pepper
2 garlic cloves, crushed
8-ounce can whole tomatoes
1 cup chickpeas, drained
1/4 cup chopped black olives

1 1/2 teaspoons chopped fresh
  rosemary, or 1/2 teaspoon dried
  rosemary, crumbled
1/4 teaspoon cinnamon
1 cup plain lowfat yogurt
1/4 cup chopped fresh mint
1/4 teaspoon salt
1/4 teaspoon freshly ground pepper
1/4 cup crumbled feta cheese

CALORIES	579
55% Carbohydrate	81 g
26% Protein	37 g
19% Fat	12 g
CALCIUM	230 mg
IRON	4 mg
SODIUM	484 mg

Preheat the oven to 300° F. Stack the pitas, wrap in foil and set aside. In a medium-size nonstick skillet, brown the lamb, onion, bell pepper and garlic over medium-high heat. Spoon into a strainer to drain fat; return to skillet. Add the tomatoes and their liquid, the chickpeas, olives, rosemary and cinnamon, stirring and mashing the chickpeas and tomatoes with a spoon, and cook until heated through. Meanwhile, heat the pitas in the oven. Combine the yogurt, mint, salt and pepper in a small bowl. Add the cheese to the skillet and heat until the cheese melts. Cut a small slice from the top of each pita. Spoon the lamb mixture into the pitas and top with the yogurt mixture.   4 servings

TABBOULEH

Whole-grain foods contain more fiber and vitamins than refined, or processed, products. When you buy bulgur (cracked wheat kernels), make sure the brown bran has not been removed.

1 cup bulgur
1 cup fresh parsley, chopped
1 cup fresh mint, chopped
1/2 cup finely chopped scallions,
  green and white parts

2 tablespoons olive oil
2 tablespoons lemon juice
1/2 teaspoon salt
2 medium tomatoes, chopped
Small head Romaine lettuce

CALORIES	291
66% Carbohydrate	48 g
10% Protein	8 g
24% Fat	8 g
CALCIUM	60 mg
IRON	4 mg
SODIUM	279 mg

Bring 2 cups of water to a boil in a small saucepan. Place the bulgur in a large bowl and pour the boiling water over it; let stand for at least 2 hours. After 2 hours, drain the bulgur well in a strainer, pressing out the excess water. Return the bulgur to the bowl, add the remaining ingredients except the lettuce and mix well. To serve, line a platter or salad bowl with lettuce leaves and mound the bulgur on top.   4 servings

Dinner

LINGUINE WITH TUNA SAUCE

Rinsing the tuna under running water reduces its sodium content.

1 tablespoon olive oil
1/4 cup chopped onion
1 garlic clove, crushed
12-ounce can crushed tomatoes
12 1/2-ounce can water-packed
   tuna, drained
1/4 cup black olives, slivered
2 tablespoons red wine

1 small bay leaf
3/4 teaspoon chopped fresh oregano,
   or 1/4 teaspoon dried oregano
1/4 teaspoon red pepper flakes
1 pound of whole-wheat or spinach
   linguine
2 tablespoons chopped fresh parsley

Heat the oil in a large saucepan. Add the onion and cook until translucent. Add the garlic and brown slightly. Add all the remaining ingredients except the linguine and parsley and bring to a boil. Reduce the heat and simmer for 20 minutes. Bring a large saucepan of water to a boil. Ten minutes before the sauce is done, cook the linguine until al dente. Drain the linguine in a colander, then transfer to 4 plates. Top with the sauce and sprinkle with chopped parsley.

4 servings

CALORIES	504
53% Carbohydrate	68 g
32% Protein	40 g
15% Fat	9 g
CALCIUM	85 mg
IRON	6 mg
SODIUM	245 mg

Linguine with Tuna Sauce

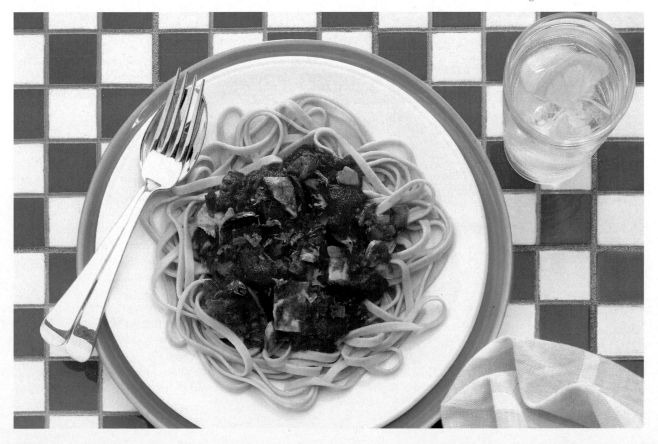

CALORIES	284
67% Carbohydrate	48 g
12% Protein	9 g
21% Fat	7 g
CALCIUM	250 mg
IRON	1 mg
SODIUM	234 mg

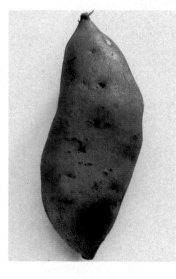

BAKED SWEET POTATOES WITH YOGURT

Sweet potatoes contain even more carbohydrates than regular potatoes and also provide substantial amounts of vitamin A.

2 cups plain lowfat yogurt
4 large sweet potatoes, about
  1/2 pound each
1 1/2 tablespoons extra-virgin olive oil

1/2 cup chopped chives
1/4 teaspoon salt
1/4 teaspoon freshly ground black
  pepper

Place the yogurt in a cheesecloth-lined strainer set over a bowl. Top with a small plate and weight with a 1-pound can. Drain for at least 1 hour.

Preheat the oven to 400° F. Wash and dry the potatoes and prick the skins with a fork. Bake the potatoes for 45 to 60 minutes, or until easily pierced with a fork. Split the cooked potatoes and top them with the drained yogurt. Drizzle olive oil over the potatoes and sprinkle them with chives, salt and pepper.

4 servings

SPINACH LASAGNA

This meatless version of lasagna is low in saturated fat because it uses skim-milk mozzarella and lowfat cottage cheese.

2 garlic cloves, crushed
1/2 pound white mushrooms,
  sliced
1 cup chopped onion
4 cups canned plum tomatoes in
  purée (two 16-ounce cans)
1 tablespoon dried basil
2 teaspoons dried oregano
2 tablespoons chopped fresh
  parsley
1/4 teaspoon salt
1/4 teaspoon freshly ground black
  pepper

1/4 teaspoon red pepper flakes
10-ounce package of whole-wheat or
  spinach lasagna noodles
Two 10-ounce packages frozen
  chopped spinach, thawed
1 tablespoon olive oil
Pinch of freshly grated nutmeg
2 cups lowfat cottage cheese (1% fat)
2 tablespoons lowfat milk (1% fat)
2 ounces part skim-milk mozzarella,
  shredded
2 tablespoons grated Parmesan
  cheese

Bring a large saucepan of water to a boil. Meanwhile, combine the garlic, mushrooms and all but 2 tablespoons of the onion in a large nonstick skillet; cover and cook over medium heat, stirring often, for about 5 minutes, or until the vegetables soften. Purée the tomatoes in a blender and add to the skillet. Add the basil, oregano, parsley, a pinch of salt and pepper and the red pepper flakes; partially cover and simmer for 30 minutes, stirring occasionally. Cook the lasagna noodles according to the package directions; set aside.

Preheat the oven to 350° F. Squeeze the excess water from the spinach. Cook the reserved onion in the oil in a nonstick skillet until softened. Add the spinach and cook, stirring, until the liquid evaporates. Add the remaining salt and pepper, and the nutmeg, and remove from the heat. Place the cottage cheese and milk in a blender and blend until smooth; set aside.

Spread a little tomato sauce on the bottom of a 9 × 13" baking dish. Form a layer using one third of the noodles, one third of the tomato sauce, half of the

CALORIES	367
56% Carbohydrate	52 g
27% Protein	24 g
17% Fat	7 g
CALCIUM	284 mg
IRON	5 mg
SODIUM	727 mg

cottage cheese, half of the spinach and half of the shredded mozzarella. Repeat with one third of the noodles and the remaining cottage cheese, mozzarella and spinach. Top with the remaining noodles, tomato sauce and the grated Parmesan. Cover loosely with foil and bake for 50 to 60 minutes, or until bubbly; remove the foil during the last 10 minutes. Let the lasagna stand for 10 minutes before serving.   6 servings

RED BEAN AND RICE SALAD

The intact bran and germ layers of brown rice provide vitamin E and fiber — both of which are missing in polished white rice.

2 tablespoons vegetable oil	1/4 cup chopped onion	
1 cup brown rice	1/4 cup chopped green bell pepper	
2 1/2 cups low-sodium chicken stock	1/4 cup chopped red bell pepper	
1 cup canned red kidney beans, rinsed and drained	1 tablespoon chopped fresh parsley	
1/4 cup sliced celery	1 tablespoon red wine vinegar	
	1/2 teaspoon hot pepper sauce	
	2 cups shredded lettuce	

CALORIES	448
65% Carbohydrate	73 g
16% Protein	19 g
19% Fat	10 g
CALCIUM	92 mg
IRON	5 mg
SODIUM	505 mg

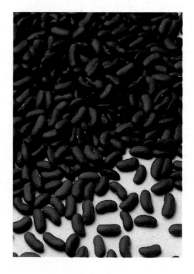

Heat 1 tablespoon of vegetable oil in a medium-size saucepan over medium-high heat. Add the rice and sauté until lightly browned. Add the chicken stock and bring to a boil. Reduce the heat and simmer the rice, covered, for 50 minutes, or until the rice is tender and the broth is completely absorbed. Drain the rice in a colander and set aside to cool for at least 30 minutes.

When cool, transfer the rice to a bowl. Add all the remaining ingredients except the lettuce and toss. Cover and refrigerate for 2 hours. To serve, line a platter with shredded lettuce and mound the salad on top.   4 servings

POTATO AND SPINACH CASSEROLE

Do not peel potatoes. The peel contains a lot of fiber and vitamins.

4 baking potatoes (about 2 pounds)	1/2 cup sliced onions
	1 1/2 cups skim milk
1/2 teaspoon minced fresh rosemary, or 1 1/2 teaspoons dried rosemary, crumbled	1 egg
	1/4 cup grated Parmesan
	1 tablespoon dry bread crumbs
2 cups fresh spinach leaves, chopped	

Preheat the oven to 350° F. Scrub and dry the potatoes and slice 1/4-inch thick. Place half of the slices in a 1 1/2-quart baking dish and sprinkle with half of the rosemary. Top the potatoes with half of the onions and spinach. Repeat the layers. Beat together the milk, egg and 3 tablespoons of the Parmesan; pour the mixture over the vegetables. Cover the dish with foil and bake for 50 minutes. Meanwhile, combine the bread crumbs with the remaining Parmesan; set aside. Remove the casserole from the oven and top with the Parmesan mixture. Return the casserole to the oven and bake, uncovered, for another 10 minutes.   4 servings

CALORIES	269
71% Carbohydrate	48 g
18% Protein	13 g
11% Fat	4 g
CALCIUM	244 mg
IRON	3 mg
SODIUM	200 mg

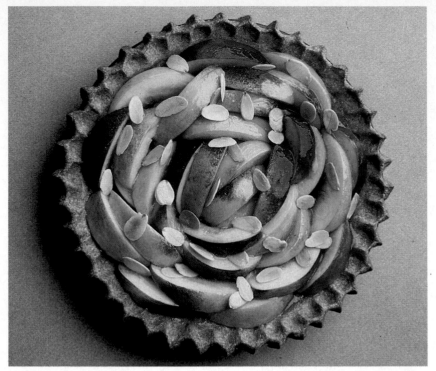

Nectarine Tart

Desserts

. . . .

NECTARINE TART

By adding extra flavor, lemon peel and lemon juice lessen the need for sugar and salt in many recipes.

1/2 cup rolled oats	1/3 cup apricot jam
1 cup sifted whole-wheat flour	1 tablespoon lemon juice
1 teaspoon grated lemon peel	4 ripe nectarines (about 1 1/2 pounds),
1/4 cup chilled margarine	cut into 1/2-inch slices
3 to 4 tablespoons ice water	2 tablespoons toasted sliced almonds

Place the oats in a blender and process to the consistency of coarse flour. In a large bowl, combine the oats, flour and lemon peel. Cut in the margarine until the mixture resembles coarse meal. Sprinkle in ice water 1 tablespoon at a time until the dough just holds together. Form the dough into a ball, flatten slightly, and wrap in wax paper. Allow the dough to rest for 10 to 15 minutes. Meanwhile, preheat the oven to 425° F.

On a lightly floured board, roll the dough into an 11-inch circle about 1/8-inch thick. Transfer the dough to a 9-inch pie plate and flute the edge. Bake the pastry shell for 12 to 15 minutes, or until lightly browned. Cool completely. Meanwhile, strain the apricot jam into a small saucepan. Add the lemon juice and cook, stirring, over low heat until the jam is thinned and warmed. Brush the inside of the pastry shell lightly with the jam, arrange the nectarine slices on top and brush with the remaining jam. Sprinkle with almonds.

6 servings

CALORIES	276
62% Carbohydrate	43 g
6% Protein	5 g
32% Fat	10 g
CALCIUM	22 mg
IRON	1 mg
SODIUM	3 mg

OATMEAL-BANANA BARS

Rolled oats contain a healthy amount of oat bran, a water-soluble fiber that aids digestion and helps lower your cholesterol level.

1 teaspoon softened margarine
2 cups rolled oats
3/4 cup whole-wheat flour
1/2 cup firmly packed light brown sugar
2 1/2 teaspoons baking powder
1/2 teaspoon cinnamon
1/4 teaspoon nutmeg
1/2 teaspoon grated orange peel

1/2 cup chopped walnuts or pecans
1/2 cup raisins
1 cup lowfat milk (1% fat)
2 eggs
1 egg white
6 tablespoons margarine, melted
3 medium-size bananas, puréed (1 1/4 cups)

CALORIES per bar	143
55% Carbohydrate	20 g
9% Protein	3 g
36% Fat	6 g
CALCIUM	39 mg
IRON	1 mg
SODIUM	92 mg

Preheat the oven to 350° F. Lightly grease a 9 × 13" baking pan, line the pan with wax paper and very lightly grease the paper. Combine the dry ingredients in a large bowl and set aside. Combine the remaining ingredients in a blender and process until smooth. Add the contents of the blender to the dry ingredients and stir to mix well. Spread the batter in the prepared pan, smoothing the top with a spatula. Bake for 25 to 30 minutes, or until the edges pull away slightly from the sides of the pan and the top is lightly browned. Place the pan on a rack to cool and then cut into bars.   Makes 24 bars

FRUIT AND NUT BRAN BREAD

Bananas are high not only in carbohydrates, but also in potassium, a mineral that is essential in the formation of muscle glycogen.

1 1/2 cups unbleached all-purpose flour
1 cup bran
1/2 cup sugar
1 teaspoon baking powder
1/2 teaspoon baking soda
1/2 cup chopped dried apricots

1/2 cup chopped toasted walnuts or hazelnuts
2 medium very ripe bananas, coarsely chopped
2 eggs, beaten
2 tablespoons safflower oil
1/3 cup orange juice
1 teaspoon vanilla extract

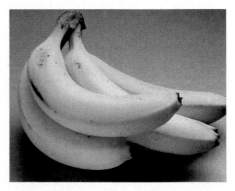

Preheat the oven to 350° F. Lightly grease a 9 × 5 × 3" loaf pan. Combine the dry ingredients in a large bowl; stir in the apricots and nuts. Add the bananas, eggs, oil, orange juice and vanilla, and mix just until blended. Pour the batter into the prepared pan and make a lengthwise cut down the center of the batter with a knife. Bake the bread for 45 minutes, or until the bread pulls away slightly from the sides of the pan. Let the bread cool in the pan 5 minutes, then turn it out onto a rack to cool completely. Wrap tightly in foil to store.

8 servings

CALORIES per 2-slice serving	306
63% Carbohydrate	48 g
8% Protein	6 g
29% Fat	10 g
CALCIUM	28 mg
IRON	2 mg
SODIUM	121 mg

Snacks

. . . .

GUACAMOLE WITH CHIPS AND CRUDITES

Corn tortillas contain almost no fat. Baking them does not add any fat the way frying does.

1 medium-size ripe avocado
1 cup lowfat cottage cheese
  (1% fat)
1 tablespoon lime juice
1 teaspoon chopped chives

1/4 to 1/2 teaspoon red pepper flakes
7-ounce package corn tortillas
2 teaspoons corn oil
Small head leaf lettuce
Assorted raw vegetables for dipping

CALORIES	179
47% Carbohydrate	21 g
18% Protein	8 g
35% Fat	7 g
CALCIUM	85 mg
IRON	2 mg
SODIUM	185 mg

Halve and peel the avocado and cut into chunks. Place in a blender with the cottage cheese, lime juice, chives and red pepper flakes; blend to the desired consistency. Refrigerate the guacamole for 2 hours.

Just before serving, preheat the oven to 400° F. Brush the tortillas lightly with oil. Cut each tortilla into 8 triangles and place on a baking sheet. Bake the tortilla triangles for 5 to 6 minutes, or until browned and crisp. Line a serving bowl with lettuce leaves and mound the guacamole on top. Serve with the tortilla chips and raw vegetables. 8 servings

Guacamole with Chips and Crudités

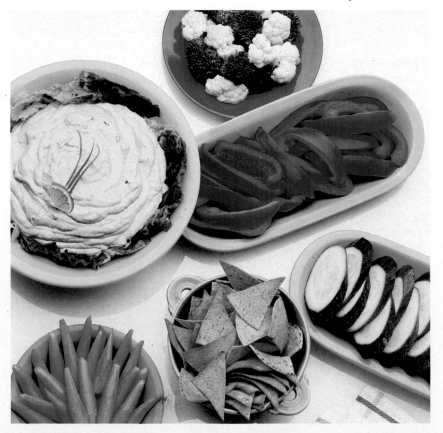

HUMMUS

Tahini, a paste made of sesame seeds, gives this Middle Eastern dish a rich, nutty taste.

20-ounce can chickpeas, drained
1/3 cup tahini
2 small garlic cloves, crushed
1/4 cup lemon juice
1/2 teaspoon ground cumin
Dash of freshly ground black
    pepper

2 tablespoons coarsely chopped fresh
    coriander or parsley
2 teaspoons olive oil
Paprika
Eight 6-inch whole-wheat pitas

CALORIES	366
58% Carbohydrate	53 g
17% Protein	16 g
25% Fat	10 g
CALCIUM	165 mg
IRON	4 mg
SODIUM	1 mg

Preheat the oven to 350° F. Combine the chickpeas, tahini, garlic, lemon juice, cumin and pepper with 1/3 cup water and 1 tablespoon of the chopped coriander or parsley in a food processor fitted with a steel blade, or in a blender, and process until the mixture is almost smooth. If the mixture is too thick, add additional water by the tablespoon. Transfer the hummus to a shallow serving bowl and drizzle with olive oil. Sprinkle with paprika and the remaining coriander or parsley.

Cut each pita into 8 wedges; separate each wedge into 2 pieces. Arrange the wedges on a baking sheet and toast in the oven for about 5 minutes, or until crisp. Serve with the hummus.   8 servings

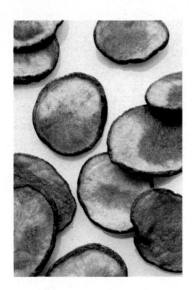

OVEN-BAKED POTATO CHIPS

You can make flavorful lowfat potato chips by baking them with a light coating of vegetable cooking spray.

1 large Idaho potato (about 3/4
    pound)

Vegetable cooking spray
Paprika

CALORIES	240
77% Carbohydrate	46 g
8% Protein	5 g
15% Fat	4 g
CALCIUM	19 mg
IRON	2 mg
SODIUM	16 mg

Preheat the oven to 400° F. Scrub the potato well and cut it crosswise into 1/8-inch-thick slices. Lightly coat a large baking sheet with cooking spray. Arrange the potato slices in one layer — overlapping them slightly if necessary — then spray the slices lightly with cooking spray. Sprinkle lightly with paprika. Bake the chips for 30 minutes, turning once, then reduce the heat to 300° F. Bake for another 15 to 20 minutes, or until the chips are crisp and brown.   1 serving

HEARTY WHOLE-WHEAT LOAF

CALORIES per slice	251
62% Carbohydrate	39 g
12% Protein	8 g
26% Fat	7 g
CALCIUM	93 mg
IRON	3 mg
SODIUM	467 mg

Whole-grain breads provide ample sources of complex carbohydrates, making them good between-meal snacks for active people.

5 1/2 cups whole-wheat flour	3/4 cup skim milk
2 cups rye flour	1/2 cup corn oil
1 cup bran	1/2 cup dark molasses
1/2 cup wheat germ	2 eggs
2 teaspoons salt	1 tablespoon cornmeal
2 packages active dry yeast	

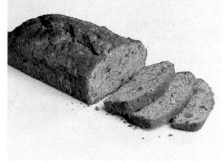

Combine 3 cups of the whole-wheat flour, the rye flour, bran and wheat germ in a large bowl. In a second large bowl combine 3 cups of this mixture with the salt and yeast. In a small saucepan combine the milk, oil, molasses and 1 cup of water. Heat over low heat until the mixture registers 120° F on a kitchen thermometer.

Gradually add the liquid mixture to the flour-yeast mixture, beating constantly with an electric mixer on low speed just until blended. Increase the speed to medium and beat for another 2 minutes. Reserving 1 egg white, beat in the remaining yolk and whole egg and an additional 2 cups of the flour mixture, and beat for another 2 minutes. Stir in the remaining flour mixture and enough additional of the whole-wheat flour to make a soft dough.

Lightly flour a countertop or board with whole-wheat flour. Turn the dough onto the floured surface and knead for about 10 minutes, or until smooth and elastic. Add more whole-wheat flour if dough is too sticky. Shape the dough into a ball and place in a greased bowl, turning the dough to grease the top. Cover and let the dough rise in a warm place for about 1 hour, or until doubled in size. Punch down the dough and turn onto a lightly floured surface. Invert the bowl over the dough and let the dough rest for another 15 minutes.

Sprinkle a baking sheet with cornmeal. Shape the dough into an oval and transfer to the baking sheet. Cover with a kitchen towel and let rise in a warm place until doubled in size.

Preheat the oven to 350° F. Cut three 1/8-inch-deep slits across the top of the loaf. Mix the reserved egg white with 1 tablespoon of water and brush the bread with the mixture. Bake the bread on the baking sheet for 50 to 60 minutes, or until the loaf sounds hollow when tapped. Remove the bread from the oven and transfer to a rack to cool. Serve the bread slightly warm, or cool it completely and wrap it tightly in foil to store.

Makes one 3-pound loaf (20 slices)

Beverages

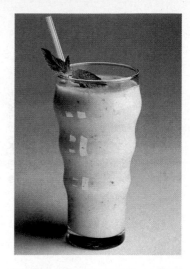

DOUBLE-HONEY DRINK

Regular milkshakes are high in fat. By including lowfat yogurt, this drink lowers the milk fat and supplies calcium plus substantial amounts of vitamins A and C from the honeydew melon.

3 cups ripe honeydew melon chunks

1 tablespoon honey

1 cup plain lowfat yogurt

2 mint sprigs, plus 4 sprigs for garnish (optional)

Combine the melon, honey, yogurt and 2 mint sprigs in a blender and purée for about 30 seconds, or until smooth. Pour into 8-ounce glasses and garnish with mint sprigs, if desired.   4 servings

CALORIES	103
78% Carbohydrate	20 g
13% Protein	3 g
9% Fat	1 g
CALCIUM	112 mg
IRON	.2 mg
SODIUM	53 mg

NONALCOHOLIC SPRITZER

You may think that drinks containing alcohol give you a lift, but they are actually depressants. Sugary alcoholic drinks are especially harmful after hot-weather exercise because they tend to raise your body temperature as well as dehydrate you. Fruit juice with sparkling water replenishes fluids lost in sweat. Drink it cold — your system will absorb the water more quickly.

3 cups white grape juice, chilled

2 cups sparkling mineral water, chilled

3 tablespoons lemon juice

Lemon twists or slices for garnish (optional)

Combine the grape juice, mineral water and lemon juice in a pitcher and stir. Serve in wineglasses and garnish with lemon twists or slices, if desired.   4 servings

CALORIES	123
95% Carbohydrate	29 g
4% Protein	1 g
1% Fat	.1 g
CALCIUM	17 mg
IRON	.5 mg
SODIUM	5 mg

BANANA SHAKE

This drink is already low in fat and high in carbohydrates, but you can raise the carbohydrate level even more by substituting fresh strawberries, peaches or nectarines for the peanut butter.

2 ripe bananas, cut into chunks

1 tablespoon natural peanut butter

2 cups skim milk

1/4 teaspoon vanilla extract

3 ice cubes

Place all of the ingredients in a blender. Blend for about 20 seconds, or until the shake is smooth and frothy.   4 servings

CALORIES	133
65% Carbohydrate	21 g
17% Protein	6 g
18% Fat	3 g
CALCIUM	181 mg
IRON	.3 mg
SODIUM	91 mg

PROP CREDITS

Page 42: shoes–Nautilus Athletic Footwear, Inc., Greenville, S.C.; pages 46-56: leotard, shoes–Reebok International LTD, Avon, Mass.; page 57: shoes–Nautilus Athletic Footwear, Inc., Greenville, S.C.; page 58: shirt, shorts, shoes: Puma USA, Inc., Framingham, Mass.; pages 64-65: shirt, shorts, shoes: Puma USA, Inc., Framingham, Mass.; pages 66-69: shirt, shorts, shoes: Nike, Inc., Beaverton, Ore.; pages 70-71: shorts, shoes–Puma USA, Inc., Framingham, Mass.; pages 72-73: shoes–Nike, Inc., Beaverton, Ore.; Athletic Style, New York City; pages 84-85: bicycle–Stuyvesant Bicycle Co., New York City; helmets–City-cycles, New York City, Stuyvesant Bicycle Co., New York City; shoes–Citycycles; pages 98-99: all equipment–The Finals, New York City; pages 112-113: all equipment–Eastern Mountain Sports, New York City; page 128: glasses–The Pottery Barn, New York City; page 131: plate–Ad Hoc Housewares, New York City; page 133: tiles–Country Floors, Inc., New York City; page 138: bowls, plates–Mood Indigo, New York City.

ACKNOWLEDGMENTS

All cosmetics and grooming products supplied by Clinique Labs, Inc., New York City.

Step-test chart (page 21) adapted from *Nutrition, Weight Control, and Exercise* by Frank I. Katch and William D. McArdle (second edition), 1983

Our thanks to Greg Avon, Isabelle Carmichael, David Carrier, Paul Daly, Ellie Hatch, Arno L. Jensen, M.D., John E. Martin, Ph.D., and Bob Vernon

Index prepared by Ian Tucker

Production by Giga Communications

PHOTOGRAPHY CREDITS

Cover: Larry Sherer; title page: Walter Iooss Jr.; pages 6-7: Rick English, *Runner's World* magazine; page 20: Dan Cunningham; page 21: Steven Mays; pages 30-31, 34-41: David Madison; pages 42-43, 46-57: Steven Mays; pages 58-59, 64-71: David Madison; pages 72-73: Steven Mays; pages 74-75, 78-82: David Epperson; pages 83-85: Steven Mays; pages 86-87, 90-97: Walter Iooss Jr.; pages 98-99: Steven Mays; pages 100-101, 104-111: Michael Kevin Daly; pages 112-113: Steven Mays; pages 114-115, 118-123: Brian Hill; pages 124-125, 128-141: Steven Mays.

ILLUSTRATION CREDITS

Page 8, chart: Brian Sisco; page 9, chart: Javier Romero, adapted with permission of the American Heart Association; page 10, chart: Brian Sisco; page 12, chart: Brian Sisco; page 16, chart: Brian Sisco, illustration: Javier Romero; page 24, charts: Brian Sisco, illustration: Javier Romero; page 25, chart: Brian Sisco; page 29, illustrations: Javier Romero; pages 34-35, illustrations: Brian Sisco; page 36, chart: Brian Sisco; page 39, illustration: Brian Sisco; page 41, illustration: Javier Romero; page 81, illustration: Javier Romero.

Time-Life Books Inc. offers a wide range of fine recordings, including a Big Band series. For subscription information, call 1-800-621-7026, or write TIME-LIFE MUSIC, Time & Life Building, Chicago, Illinois 60611.

Achilles tendon, 71
aerobic exercise, 6-17
    age and, 11, 12-14
    amount of, 8
    appetite and, 19
    body fat and, 12
    cancer and, 17
    cardiovascular system and, 7-9
    vs. diet, for weight loss, 12
    energy sources during, 10, 13
    heart attacks and, 15-17
    heart rate and, see heart rate
    injuries from, see injuries
    longevity and, 16, 17
    muscle-fiber types and, 13
    pollution and, 14
    during pregnancy, 13
    program of, see aerobic exercise
        program
    psychological effects of, 11-12, 14
    sexuality and, 15
    stopping, effects of, 14
    stress and, 12
    sudden death and, 16-17
    types of, see aerobic movement; cross-
        country skiing; cycling; rowing; run-
        ning; swimming; walking
aerobic exercise program, 18-29
    choosing an exercise, 23
    cool-down, 25, 28
    cross-training and, 23, 26
    exercise levels, 26-27
    fitness assessment, 18-21
    pacing, 25
    staying with it, 23
    stretching routine, 28, 29
    warm-up, 25, 28
aerobic movement, 23, 43-57
    arm exercises, 48-49, 55
    cool-down, 56
    fitness benefits of, 43-44
    injuries from, 14, 44-45
    jumping rope, 57
    leg exercises, 51-55
    low-impact, 45
    program tips, 45
    routine for, 46-56
    shoes for, 44
    torso exercises, 50
    warm-up, 46-47
age, aerobic exercise and, 12, 14-15
alignment, in running, 69
anaerobic exercise, 8, 10
appetite, 19
arms, aerobic movement exercises for,
    48-49
ATP (adenosine triphosphate), 10

Beginning exercise level, 27
beverage recipes, 129, 141
bicycles, 75-76, 84, 85
    see also cycling
blood pressure, 15, 19, 28, 127
body fat, 12, 13, 18
breakfast recipes, 128-129
breathing, 67, 93
brisk walking, 32, 34, 36, 41

Cadence, in cycling, 81
calcium
    amounts in recipe dishes, 128-141
    supplements, 127
calories, 126-141
    amounts in recipe dishes, 128-141
    conversion to grams, 127
    recommended nutrient proportions
        for, 127
    walking and, 36
cancer, and exercise, 17, 127
carbohydrate loading, 127
carbohydrates, 125-141
    amounts in recipe dishes,
        128-141
    endurance and, 13, 60, 125-126
    types of, 126
cardiovascular system, 7-9
    see also heart rate
carriage, in running, 66-67
cholesterol, 15-16, 19, 27,
        97
    fiber and, 19
clothes
    for cross-country skiing, 102-103
    for cycling, 77
    for running, 60, 62
    for walking, 33
competitive exercise level, 27
complex carbohydrates, 126
cool-down, 25, 28, 56
CP (creatine phosphate), 10
crawl stroke, 90-95
cross-country skiing, 23, 101-113
    clothes for, 102-103
    diagonal stride in, 104-106
    double poling in, 107
    downhill technique in, 110
    equipment for, 112-113
    fitness benefits of, 101-102
    injuries from, 102
    program tips, 103
    skating in, 108
    uphill technique in, 110
cross-training, 23, 26
cuboid bone displacement, 71

cycling, 23, 26, 75-85
    bicycles for, 75-76, 84, 85
    cadence in, 81
    clothing for, 77
    fitness benefits of, 76
    gearing in, 81
    handlebars, gripping, 82-83
    hazards in, 76
    helmets for, 76, 84
    hills and, 77, 80
    injuries from, 77
    posture in, 79
    program tips, 77
    stationary indoor, 76

Dessert recipes, 136-137
diet
    vs. aerobic exercise, for weight
        loss, 12
    running and,
    see also carbohydrates;
        recipes
dinner recipes, 133-135

Endorphins, 60-61
energy sources during exercise, 10, 13
    see also carbohydrates
exercise, see aerobic exercise;
    anaerobic exercise

Fast-twitch muscle fiber, 13
fat, body, 12, 13, 18
fat, dietary, 126
    amounts in recipe dishes, 128-141
    cholesterol and, 19
    recommended dietary intake of, 127
fitness level, assessment of, 18-21
fitness measurement, see VO$_2$max
Fixx, Jim, 16-17
fluid replacement, 61, 89
food, 10, 13
    see also carbohydrates;
        diet; recipes
footstrike, 67, 68

Glucose, 10, 126
grams, conversion of calories to, 127
groin, stretching exercise for, 29

Hamstrings, stretching
    exercise for, 29
HDL cholesterol, 27
heart, 7-9

heart attacks, 15-17
heart rate
 aerobic movement and, 44
 effect of exercise on, 9, 11
 maximum, 25
 pulse taking, 21, 25
 resting, 8, 11
 swimming and, 88
 target, 24, 25
 walking and, 31, 36
hip rotation, in race walking, 40-41
hormones, 60-61
hypertension, 15, 19, 127

Iliotibial band friction
 syndrome, 71
injuries, 14, 23
 from aerobic movement, 14, 44-45
 from cross-country skiing, 102
 from cycling, 77
 from rowing, 116
 from running, 63, 70-71
insulin, 126
iron
 amounts in recipe dishes, 128-141
 supplements, 127

Jogging in place, 47, 56
joints, 14
jumping rope, 57

LDL cholesterol, 19
legs
 aerobic movement exercises for, 51-55
 stretching exercises for, 29
longevity, 16, 17
low-impact aerobics, 45
lunch recipes, 130-132

Marathon runners, 11, 13, 15, 60
muscle development, 12
 cross-country skiing and, 102
 cycling and, 76
 rowing and, 115
 swimming and, 87-88
muscle fibers, types of, 13
muscles, 8-10

National Institutes of Health, 127
neck, stretching exercise for, 29

Optimum exercise level, 27

Paffenbarger, Ralph S., 15-17
peak exercise level, 27
plantar fascitis, 70
poles, ski, 113

pollution, 14
polyunsaturated fats, 19
posture
 in cycling, 79
 in walking, 34, 35, 38
pregnancy, 13
protein
 amounts in recipe dishes, 128-141
 recommended dietary intake of, 127
psychological effects of
 aerobic exercise, 11-12, 14
pulse taking, 21, 25

Race walking, 32, 38-41
reaction time, 12
recipes
 beverage, 129, 141
 breakfast, 128-129
 dessert, 136-137
 dinner, 133-135
 lunch, 130-132
 snack, 138-140
relaxation, 18-19
rowing, 23, 115-121
 balance in, 119
 fitness benefits of, 115-116
 program tips, 117
 stroke in, 119-121
 weather and, 116-117
rowing machines, 116
rowing shells, 116, 117,
 122-123
runner's high, 60-61
runner's knee, 71, 77
running, 23, 26, 59-73
 alignment in, 69
 carriage in, 66-67
 clothes for, 60, 62
 diet and, 60
 fitness benefits of, 60
 fluid replacement and, 61
 footstrike in, 67, 68
 genetic predisposition for, 59-60
 injuries from, 63, 70-71
 program tips, 63
 psychological benefits of, 60-61
 shoes for, 61-62, 72-73
 stride in, 65
 surfaces for, 62
 weather and, 62-63

Saddle height, in cycling, 79
sciatic pain, 71
sexuality, 15
shin splints, 32, 44, 71
shoes
 for aerobic movement, 44
 for cycling, 77
 for running, 61-62, 72-73
 for walking, 33
simple carbohydrates, 126

skating, in cross-country
 skiing, 108-109
skiing, see cross-country skiing
slow-twitch muscle fibers, 13
snack recipes, 138-140
sodium
 amounts in recipe dishes, 128-141
 recommended dietary intake of, 127
starches, 10, 126
stationary indoor cycling, 76
step test, 20-21
stress, 12
stretching, 28, 29, 56
stride
 in cross-country skiing, 104-106
 in running, 65
striding, 32, 35, 36
stroke, rowing, 119-121
stroke rating, 117
sugars, 126
swimming, 23, 26, 87-99
 aids to, 98-99
 ailments related to, 96, 97
 breathing during, 93
 crawl stroke, 90-95
 eating before, 89
 fitness benefits of, 87-88
 fluid replenishment and, 89
 heart rate and, 88
 pools for, 88
 program tips, 89
 pyramids in, 89

Tendinitis, 77
torso, aerobic movement exercises for, 50
"training effect," 8

VO₂max, 11, 13, 15, 23
 aerobic movement and, 44
 cross-country skiing and, 102
 running and, 60
 swimming and, 87
 walking and, 31, 36

Walking, 23, 31-41
 brisk, 32, 34, 36, 41
 clothes for, 33
 fitness benefits of, 31
 hill training, 36
 program tips, 33
 race, 32, 38-41
 shoes for, 33
 striding, 32, 35, 36
 with weights, 36, 37
warm-up, 25, 28, 46-47
weather
 cycling and, 76
 rowing and, 116-117
 running and, 62-63
weight reduction, 12, 13, 19